PRECOR PRESENTS:

Alberto Salazar

THE **TREADMILL TRAINING**

AND **WORKOUT GUIDE**

PRECOR PRESENTS:

Alberto Salazar

THE
TREADMILL
TRAINING
AND
WORKOUT
GUIDE

Alberto Salazar & Len Sherman

HATHERLEIGH PRESS • *New York, New York*

A GETFITNOW.COM BOOK

Hatherleigh Press/Getfitnow.com Books
An Affiliate of W.W. Norton & Company, Inc.
5-22 46th Avenue Suite 200
Long Island City, NY 11101
1-212-832-1584

Visit our website:
www.getfitnow.com

DISCLAIMER: Before beginning any exercise program consult your physician. The authors and publisher of this book and workout disclaim any liability, personal or professional, resulting from the misapplication of any of the training procedures described in this publication.

All Getfitnow.com titles are available for bulk purchase, special promotions, and premiums. For more information, please contact the manager of our Special Sales Department at 1-800-528-2550.

Library of Congress Cataloging-in-Publication Data

Salazar, Alberto, 1958–
    Precor presents Alberto Salazar, the treadmill training and workout guide /
    Alberto Salazar & Len Sherman
        p.   cm.
    ISBN 1-57856-080-9 (alk. paper)
        1. Exercise—Equipment and supplies. 2. Running—Training. I. Title: Alberto Salazar, the treadmill training and workout guide. II. Title: Treadmill training and workout guide. III. Sherman, Len, 1956– IV. Title.
    GV543.S24 2000
    613.7'172—dc21   00-028124
                                                                          CIP

Cover design by Lisa Fyfe
Text design and composition by John Reinhardt Book Design
Principle photography by Peter Field Peck with Canon® cameras and lenses
on Fuji® print and slide film

Printed in Canada on acid-free paper

10 9 8 7 6 5 4 3 2 1

ACKNOWLEDGMENTS

APART FROM THOSE WHO HELD THE KEYBOARDS in their hands and tapped out the words, Jeanine Rossell of Precor deserves the most applause for directing this book to completion. She guided the process from beginning to end, navigating past some turbulent shoals. Simply put, without her enthusiasm and talent, there would be no book.

A word of thanks also belongs to Andrew Flach and Kevin Moran of Hatherleigh Press.

Separately and together, their vision and skill made them the right publishers for this work.

In the end, this book is nothing more or less than the experience and ideas of its contributors, and we have been lucky to assemble a distinguished lot:

Jeff Galloway has led runners everywhere to new awareness and success through his innovative techniques, which he has generously shared here. His training methods, found in these pages, have already served to alter perception and reality for untold thousands of runners.

In addition, the contributions of trainers Isabel Lorca and Paul Frediani, Olympic gold medalist Nikki Stone, chef Chris Bianco and nutritionist Stephanie Jenkins have provided lessons and examples that reach far beyond the treadmill.

Contents

Prologue

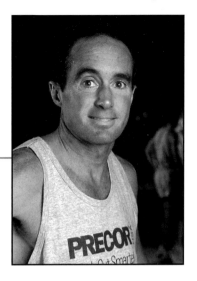

FROM BEGINNER TO PROFESSIONAL, I've been a runner for more than a quarter century. Though running is as much a daily habit to me as brushing my teeth, it is much more than a routine—it also is a cherished part of my life. The truth is, if I don't get my run in every day, I just don't feel right.

Unlike the vast majority of people who lace up their sneakers and regularly exercise, running has been more than simply recreational for me, it has been my career. Even so, the motivation behind my running has changed—evolved, you might say—quite a bit through the years. Instead of running primarily to prepare myself for competition, I now run—as well as walk and cross train—because I enjoy it, and because I want to stay healthy. Exercise provides me with an hour or so when I can be alone and reflect on the day ahead. After running, I always feel relaxed and ready to go to work. Despite its physical demands, running is an enjoyable and exhilarating activity that I always look forward to.

Running is a priority for me, so I make sure I get it in first thing in the morning. The way I figure it, all the challenges and problems at the office and at home will still be waiting for me, but my physical and mental health may not be optimal if I don't first do my training.

I began to run when I was a high school freshman in Massachusetts back in 1972, after being inspired by my older brother, who was a very good high school and college runner. He used to organize all the kids in the neighborhood to run sprints on the sidewalk, or race around the block. I didn't train but would run in these races a couple of times a week, New England weather permitting.

I was young, didn't know about training or schedules. I ran because it was fun! There was no pressure. I ran when I wanted to, and didn't run if I wasn't in the mood.

That's the way any child will approach a sport, on the basis of the question: Is this fun? Often when adults get involved and regulate the activity, making it something very different from its original intent, it is no longer enjoyable and the child will stop the activity. Lesson to one and all, regardless of age: Running needs to be enjoyable, or you won't keep doing it no matter how great its benefits.

By the time I was a junior in high school, I had become a state high school champion. I set a world age group record for a 16-year-old in the 5000 meters after finishing second in the National Junior Championships, competing against kids who were 19-year-old college freshmen. After that race, my goals and motivation for running started to change gradually from just having fun and trying to better my times, to moving up the ladder against the best runners in the country.

My grades were good and my running was constantly improving, so when the time came, I was able to attend any college in the country. I chose the University of Oregon because at the time it was pre-eminent for distance runners. While there I became an NCAA champion and even won my first try at the marathon distance in the 1980 New York City Marathon. I set a world record in New York, for a first attempt at the marathon. By my graduation in 1981, I ran the marathon in 2:08:13, breaking a 13-year world record by 19 seconds.

Though running was still fun, it was also very stressful and pressure-filled. I was always expected to win or run a fast time so I was always pondering my next workout or race, and worrying if my training wasn't proceeding exactly as planned. Running was mainly about competition for me and my satisfaction with it depended solely on my performance in my races. Not very healthy or fun! In fact, only later after several years in retirement, was I finally able to stop worrying about running fast. I recaptured some of the freedom and joy I felt when I was a boy running around the block, and really started to enjoy running again.

In late 1994, while running, I stepped into a hole and ruptured a tendon in the side of my foot, which began a five-year period of injuries and several operations. Finally, after complete reconstructive foot surgery in early 1999, I am once again completely healthy and training hard . . . but making sure to keep it fun this time around.

Before I became injured, I realized that my age (I was in my mid-thirties) had rendered my body unable to stand the impact and stresses of running all my mileage on hard pavement. I started to experiment with training on a treadmill, from walking to running to cross training. I researched all the treadmills on the market in order to decide which would be the best treadmill to have in my home. I had about three different treadmills sent to my house for my personal testing sessions. I ended up choosing a Precor treadmill because I felt, and still believe, that it provides the best cushioning, smoothness and responsiveness.

> The treadmill is used by everyone, including the top runners in the world, seeking to gain that vital, extra edge.

Precor has a patented technology that allows you to run on a perfectly flat belt that responds to every slight change in your speed and weight, thus absorbing shock and providing an exceptionally smooth run. Prior to my foot injury in 1994, I did over half of my weekly 120 miles of training on my treadmill to prepare for the most prestigious ultra-marathon in the world, the 54-Mile Comrades Marathon in South Africa. It was my first race ever further than the traditional 26.2 mile marathon distance, and my treadmill training prepared me so well that I shocked all the skeptics by winning.

I've run over 10,000 miles on my current treadmill, and, apart from replacing the belt 1,000 miles ago, the machine has never required any major maintenance, and has never needed repair. Other Precor cross training machines that I have used as part of my training are the EFX Elliptical Fitness Crosstrainer, the Stretch Trainer, and Stairclimber. All three have been trouble-free.

During the good weather months here in Oregon, I now use my treadmill about three times a week to do my faster running. When it turns colder and wetter, I will run four to five times each week indoors on the treadmill. Running this often on the treadmill has definitely helped me stay healthier by cutting down on the excessive pounding on the streets.

After all my experience running, and all my experience on the treadmill, I was very excited by the opportunity to help Precor with this book. The goal of this book is to provide guidance in using the treadmill as a basic training device to a wide range of people—from beginners, to those who have tried and failed to stick to a walking program, to good runners who want to be better. And have no doubt—*the treadmill is used by everyone, including the top runners in the world, seeking to gain that vital, extra edge.*

When I was 16, I was most fortunate to start training with the Greater Boston Track Club, which was coached by the eminent Bill Squires. Squires' most famous pupil at the time was Bill Rodgers, then the best marathoner in the world, who would win the New York City and Boston Marathons four times each.

As the only teenager at the track club, I was exposed to world-class training methods and theory at a very early age. Although my workouts were scaled back from what Bill Rodgers was doing, the principles remained the same. Being thrust into such elite company gave me tremendous confidence and motivation to work hard. It is one thing to do the right training—it is just as important to believe that it will work. The proper mental attitude will make your training not only easier but also vastly more effective. It is this belief in yourself and in your training that often means the difference between achieving and not achieving your goals. This book is intended to give the reader both the knowledge and the confidence to train correctly, and to understand exactly what the training should accomplish. It has been proven that positive thinking often leads to good results while negative thinking leads to the opposite. Nonetheless, positive thinking can only come from having the required information and tools to allow you to plan reasonably and act well.

In other words, if you don't know what you're doing, or don't know why you're supposed to be doing it, it is very difficult to possess and project an assertive, assured attitude.

The principles of both physical and mental conditioning apply to a 2:08 marathoner as well as a 4-hour-plus marathoner. Of course the actual workouts need to be adjusted to allow for skills, goals, and other factors. Nevertheless, the same fundamental principles always apply.

Within these pages, you will discover the power to train as intelligently as the best athletes in the world, while you adjust for your current level of fitness, your background, and your ambitions. Knowing that you are training smartly and safely will make your exercise program easier, more enjoyable and definitely more productive.

In this brief prologue, I have concentrated on running, because that's been my life. Your athletic interests and exercise goals might lie elsewhere; you might want to develop a walking program with plenty of hill work, or cross train, incorporating squats and lunges and the Precor EFX Elliptical Fitness Crosstrainer. Whatever your goal, this book will help you attain it more safely, quickly, and effectively than you might have imagined.

Have confidence in what you're about to read. Believe in it, take it to heart, and chances are you will attain your goals. After that, all you have to do is lace up your shoes, turn on the treadmill and start MOVING!

Alberto Salazar
November 17, 1999

Introduction

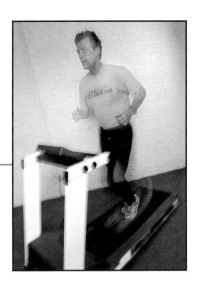

WALK INTO A BOOKSTORE these days and you can't help but notice that fitness books constitute the hottest category, overflowing the shelves. Virtually all of these books make extraordinary promises: Learn the exercise secrets known only to grand master ninjas living in monasteries somewhere west of Shangri-La; swim the dolphin way and gain not only optimal conditioning but also gills; or, more simply, pogo till your muscles pop.

This book is different. We have assembled a group of experts to explain, step by step what you realistically need to do to attain the level of fitness you seek by using a treadmill. Walking, running, cross training—the pros provide their best techniques and programs to get you motivated and moving. And, if you read carefully and follow their advice, you will get into better shape.

Many of you will exclaim, "Thank you, that's just what I wanted! Give me the formula, the prescription, and let me go at it!"

But there is much more to exercising. Exercise is more than simply moving one foot after the other. It is also about having fun, eating better and feeling stronger, more limber and alert. It is about appreciating and enjoying every moment of your life.

That is what exercise can bring you—fitness of mind and spirit, as well as body. There are no miracles, wonder drugs or machines that do the work for you. You must take charge and change your life so that you can do all that you want to do and experience all you wish to experience.

No group of people understands these exhilarating possibilities better than the people at Precor. Precor designs and manufactures some of the finest exercise equipment on the market, and we know how users of our treadmills and other equipment can gain the most from our machines.

That is why we developed this book, and asked some of the most respected athletes and trainers in the sports business to get involved. We want to ensure that you use your treadmill in a way that takes the most advantage of its capabilities, and maximizes the benefit to you.

This book focuses on the treadmill as the primary training tool to accomplish all the aforementioned fitness goals. Unfailingly dependable and surprisingly versatile, the treadmill works for anyone and everyone, regardless of age, ability or fitness level.

It surely can work for you.

CHAPTER 1
Health and Fitness: The Elusive Goal

HEALTH AND FITNESS: everybody wants it, everybody needs it—and some of us actually endeavor to gain it. *Health and Fitness* is a phrase that has been repeated so frequently and so insistently, in medical journals on TV talk shows, in exercise classes and physicians' offices, that it has been burned into our collective consciousness. It has become a single idea, one overwhelming sentiment.

Despite the increased awareness and discussion of the important role that exercise plays in maintaining and improving our health and fitness, we find ourselves in a national crisis. Studies reveal that most Americans are losing the battle of the bulge, as well as the cholesterol conflict, the flexibility fight, the wellness war, the . . . well, you get the idea.

Regardless, we keep trying—or at least keep talking about trying. Spurred by athleticism or anxiety, frustration or fear, dedication or despair, we buy memberships to mirror-filled gyms in record numbers, purchase tons of gleaming home fitness equipment, and acquire thick books filled with gorgeous photography of perfectly proportioned men and women pushing metal weights and jumping over plastic steps.

Unfortunately, studies show that the majority of people stop going to their mirror-filled gyms after only a few weeks, cease using their home exercise equipment, and quit reading those thick books, shoving them into the back of the closet, where they sit for generations, the papers yellowing, eventually deteriorating.

That's why we're here, to make sense of all the information and all the hype, and to help you make the most of your time and effort, so you can achieve your fitness goals.

As you can tell from its title, this book focuses on cardiovascular training via the treadmill. Presumably, this subject holds some appeal for you as well.

We will use Precor equipment to illustrate our plans and programs, when equipment is required for the sake of example. However, the tips and lessons provided here will work on any company's equipment — assuming, naturally enough, that the other company's treadmill is reasonably reliable.

Basics Of Aerobic Exercise

Exercise comes in many forms. The truth is, just about any time you engage in physical activity, just about any time you move your feet and your arms, just about any time you get your heart rate up, you're doing your body some good.

That is not to say that all exercise is created equal. Some types of exercise are more efficient and effective than others are in achieving specific goals, or attaining health and fitness.

Basically, exercise falls into two categories: anaerobic and aerobic. Anaerobic (translated from Latin meaning *without oxygen*) refers to exercise that is of high intensity and short duration, geared primarily to promote muscular-skeletal fitness. Carbohydrates are utilized for energy during anaerobic exercise.

Anaerobic training, such as strength or weight training, pays terrific dividends in many ways. Lifting weights improves your metabolic rate, as well as strengthens your muscles and protects your joints, back, and other vulnerable parts of your body. Weight training is particularly advantageous for women because it can help prevent osteoporosis, a condition where the bones weaken and become brittle. And, of course, increased strength can make life more enjoyable in a variety of ways: from making it easier to lift a package or a baby, to providing a sense of satisfaction when you look in the mirror.

Aerobic training (*with oxygen*) refers to the sort of continuous, usually moderate-to-intense exercise that is done to maintain cardiovascular fitness and health. Oxygen, carbohydrates and fat are the fuels burned during aerobic exercise. (For the purposes of this book, cardio training —the exercise of the cardiovascular system, and aerobic training—the method by which cardio exercise is undertaken—will be used interchangeably.)

Without a doubt, aerobic conditioning is a central component of an effective exercise program. Aerobic conditioning done for 20–30 minute sessions empowers the muscles and organs most vital to our well-being: It fortifies the heart and lungs, strengthens the legs and abdominals, and increases the level of oxygen in the blood.

Studies consistently show the lifelong benefits of being aerobically fit. These benefits extend to every area of life, from strengthening your heart to reducing your cholesterol levels to increasing your flexibility, all of which adds up to feeling, working and playing better. Furthermore, in 1996 the Surgeon General of the United States released a report that linked aerobic exercise with the prevention of several serious chronic diseases such as heart disease, stroke, diabetes and cancer.

> Aerobic exercise (has been linked) with the prevention of several serious chronic diseases such as heart disease, stroke, diabetes and cancer.

All of these benefits, and we haven't even mentioned losing weight!

You want to burn calories? Get up and run! (Or get up and walk, if you prefer.) Study after study confirms the self-evident: Running on a treadmill works as well as, and often more efficiently, than other forms of aerobic exercise. Universities and research groups have repeatedly conducted tests using a variety of stationary aerobic equipment, to compare the efficacy of treadmills, cross-country ski machines, exercise bikes, and aerobic riders in burning calories. Reports by the *Journal of the American Medical Association*, the American College of Sports Medicine, the University of New Mexico, the Medical College of Wisconsin, and a number of other institutes and groups, come to the same conclusion. Regardless of an individual's gender, height, weight or fitness level, treadmills burn more calories per hour than other devices. These studies demonstrate the supremacy of the treadmill for exercise.

The number of people who rely on the treadmill for their primary exercise is absolutely astonishing. According to the Fitness Products Council and America Sports Data Inc., Americans recently spent $1.6 billion on treadmills for their homes. Consider the following statistics on the increasing popularity of treadmills: in 1987, 4.4 million Americans exercised on a treadmill, whether at home or in a gym. Ten years later, in 1997, that figure had exploded to over 36 million Americans.

Clearly, many people are using treadmills. However, how many are getting the most from their efforts? And how many still have a thing or two to learn?

That's why we're here.

Let's Begin

In this book we cover many different topics. We provide some of the best plans for seasoned exercisers who want to engage in more productive walking or running, and are ready to increase their mileage or speed.

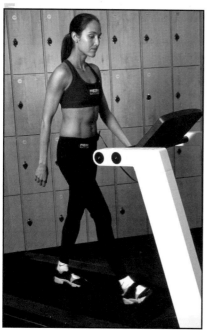

We also talk to beginners who are just looking for some help getting started. We discuss training for specific activities, such as marathons, for beginner or expert.

We hit on related subjects, such as nutrition and stretching, and demonstrate some exercises that can only be done on a treadmill. And, we hop off the treadmill for a moment to touch on the latest advancement in the mechanics of aerobic training, the Precor EFX Elliptical Fitness Crosstrainer, and how it might fit into your exercise routine.

And, if all this talk about treadmill training encourages you to clear away a corner in your bedroom and take a trip to your local exercise equipment store, we provide a quick primer on how to choose a machine that is right for you.

Overall, we want to inspire you to get on a treadmill and enjoy both the experience and the benefits of a treadmill workout. Inspiration is tricky, because all of us respond to different emotional and environmental triggers. Despite that, some realities are universal.

Just as aerobic training can benefit virtually everyone — couch potato and ultra-marathoner, male and female, young and old— this book can benefit all who seek some fitness guidance. As a reader you also may gain some wisdom along the way, because between the facts and statistics, the plans and programs, we hear the stories and experiences of some extremely accomplished athletes who have dreamed and labored — sometimes suffered and endured — and finally emerged triumphant, at times even beyond their own imaginations. We listen to their stories hoping to gain some insight into our own struggles and dreams.

> **Exercise isn't only about working and competing — it's also about having fun.**

In the end, the mission of this book is simple and straightforward: Whether your individual championship dreams are locked onto a vision of having the strength and stamina for that final kick in the Olympic 1500, or gutting it out in the last round in the club squash tournament, or simply having the legs to run up and down the sidelines as you coach your kid's soccer team, our purpose is to provide you with some of the tools you will need to pursue those dreams.

And perhaps you will find that you even go beyond your own expectations. Perhaps you will find that running once or twice around the block no longer satisfies you. Perhaps you will find yourself motivated to run longer and harder. Perhaps, eventually, you will find yourself deep in the midst of that immense pack of excited runners on the Verrazano Bridge on a crisp November morning, jogging in place to keep your limbs loose and warm, waiting for the cannon to sound the start of the annual New York City Marathon.

On the other hand, perhaps not. Perhaps being able, finally, to run around the block without feeling winded, sick and dizzy will be sufficient, and immensely gratifying.

Whatever your personal fitness goal, the treadmill will help you discover your preferences and unleash your potential. Where that eventually takes you will be up to you, and what you discover about yourself as you walk, run and train.

Before we begin remember one thing: exercise isn't only about working and competing — it's also about having fun. It's about playing and feeling good and laughing and, once again, because it cannot be said too often, having fun. So as we go through the ins-and-outs, the ups-and-downs, of treadmill training, try to save a piece of yourself to savor the moments you spend on the treadmill.

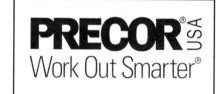

David Smith, founder of Precor had a saying that sums up the ultimate philosophy of this book: "Work Out Smarter." Yes. Exactly. You can be sure we'll return to that phrase, again and again.

So let's start reading. Let's start considering our goals and desires, our options and possibilities.

This opening chapter began with a short phrase and that's how it ends:

Let's start enjoying . . .

CHAPTER 2

The Power of Knowledge

THE KEY TO EXERCISING EFFICIENTLY and effectively is information. Information leads to awareness, and awareness to understanding. If you understand something you are able to extract the most from a situation and can respond and adapt to mistakes, changes and unanticipated events. When exercising, you need knowledge to maximize your workout and prevent injury.

Let's run through a few of the basics of running.

The number one problem runners encounter — aside from repetition and boredom, which are very dogged issues for many — is the prospect of injury. The typical runner strikes the ground with three to five times his body weight, placing considerable stress on his muscles, joints, ligaments, cartilage, etc. The surface upon which the runner lands therefore, becomes a crucial factor as to whether he or she will suffer pain or injury.

One of the studies Precor relied upon when designing its treadmill indicated that the impact that the runner absorbs when landing on the ground and whatever jarring, shock and pain is transmitted in that instant, is instantly converted in the runner's mind into *work*. The more jarring, shock and pain felt by the runner, the greater the amount of work the runner believes he is doing.

For Precor, one of the answers to building a better treadmill was obvious: Include more cushioning to absorb the impact, and the runner experiences less work and injury.

Let's talk about running surfaces that aren't cushioned, starting with the most damaging and difficult.

Nothing is harder on the legs than unforgiving cement sidewalks. If you have to run in the heart of the big city, choose the asphalt streets over the cement sidewalks.

Grass is dramatically softer, and thus gentler on the body, but its uneven surface poses other hazards. Take a wrong step, even if the level plane is off by just a few degrees, and you may twist your ankle or wrench your knee, resulting in potentially severe damage.

Soft sand is usually thought of as a terrific place to run because it is yielding and safe. How many people hurried to the beach after watching "Chariots of Fire," and the memorable scene of the English lads dashing in slow motion through the surf, laughing, splashing, training, theme music playing in the background? Despite the allure of running with the wind in your hair, the sun in your face, and sand in your shoes, be careful. Soft sand causes the heel, which normally lands first, to sink in much more deeply than when running on a solid surface, which means that it takes that much more effort to pull it out and upward. This can result in tremendous strain on the heel, and specifically on the Achilles Tendon.

And that's not all. The knee can easily be strained or twisted when pulling out of the sand, and if the Achilles Tendon and the knee are endangered, the rest of the leg is vulnerable as well.

The best surface is generally thought to be a dirt and cinder track: even and pliable, fast and safe. However, such tracks are not always easy to find, and then there is the dilemma of rain, sleet and snow, when even the best of surfaces are rendered unusable.

Then there's the treadmill. Seems a simple enough situation: belt moving one way, you moving the other. As with most interesting things in life, it's not. And the better you understand what's going on with the technology of the treadmill, the better you'll be able to maximize capabilities and get the most from your training.

Complications begin not with the machine but with the human body. Though it may appear that a person in the process of walking or running is progressing at a constant speed, in reality the feet are actually speeding up and slowing down throughout each stride. When the heel strikes the ground, the foot slows down, until it comes to a near complete stop by the time the sole is mostly flat upon the surface. To compensate for this deceleration the foot undergoes considerable acceleration when lifting off the ground.

This entire operation, repeated each time anyone takes a step, whether walking or running, takes only microseconds, and serves to protect our bodies—especially our joints—from the damaging effects of continually banging back down to earth, with the three to five times body weight impact previously mentioned.

These constant changes in foot speed are key to understanding the treadmill. If you are moving in this slow-fast manner, and the treadmill is moving at a different, steady pace, the result can be a series of conflicting, confusing signals in your brain. Expressed another way, the sensation can feel like you are running on ice: unsteady, unsure, unsafe.

That's why most treadmill manufacturers try to incorporate some means of compensating for this discrepancy.

Precor's unique solution is called Integrated Footplant Technology (IFT) and was devised 20 years ago by David Smith to coordinate the timing between foot and machine. Here's how it works:

The system replicates the alterations in the user's foot speed that occur with each step. A sensor on the treadmill's motor alerts the electronic software to speed up or slow down, instantly calculating walking or running speed, along with weight or force of the exerciser. This calculation is expressed by the software sending "power bits," expressed in algorithms, along to make subtle adjustments. The process occurs too rapidly to be consciously observed; rather, its effectiveness can be felt as the belt beneath the runner's feet moves in a smooth, safe and apparently effortless manner.

This information should help you know what to expect from a treadmill's mechanism, allowing you to physically and mentally prepare for your workout. That knowledge and preparation constitute the essence of "working out smarter." Perhaps this sounds like much ado about nothing. And if you happen to be using the treadmill to simply walk slowly forward, then this information might have limited value.

To a certain degree, slow walking is slow walking, and there's only so much you can do to change or affect that. However, as you get into running, and start moving faster, as well as uphill and downhill, and add in a few tricks that we're going to teach you — including walking sideways and backward—every bit of data you can collect might prove the difference between success and failure.

Beyond running surfaces, much of what you need to know about safe running is common sense. Whether you're lacing on brand-new running shoes for the first time, or whether you long ago bronzed the sneakers in which you set the world steeplechase record, you have to function as your own coach/trainer/physician/psychologist. Always listen to both your body and your mind, and know when to press and when to lighten up.

Here are a handful of tips that might prove useful to you as you work out:

1 Be reasonable and realistic. Gyms and health clubs thrive off people who walk in the door all excited about working hard and getting into shape, and who sign up for a three-year membership only to drop out after only a few weeks because they got frustrated, bored or injured. One gym chain privately estimates that 75 percent of new members rarely if ever show up to exercise after the first three weeks. (That's why your local gym never, _ever_ stops selling memberships — and the place somehow maintains its daily traffic _status quo_. It's kind of like that trick where the circus clowns keep piling into the little car, but never seem to fill it up.)

When you start an exercise program, start reasonably, with achievable objectives that are not overwhelming. Why?

Imagine that you are about to begin running your first marathon. Because of the intensity of that moment, it is virtually impossible not to reflect on how very far you have to go. The thought of facing all those city blocks, avenues and bridges, all those water stops and medical checkpoints, all the fatigue, blisters and cramps, while you're still working your way through Mile One, can quickly become overwhelming, causing you to falter psychologically long before your body faces any real physical challenges. Instead, concentrate on finishing that first mile. That's all. That's enough. Rejoice in that accomplishment for a while, and then focus on the next mile. Keep going, keep pumping your arms and moving your legs. Enjoy your little victories, and at the end of the race, you'll have run an entire marathon.

Similarly, the novice exerciser shouldn't pledge to work out three hours a day, seven days a week. Rather, three to four days a week for a half-hour at a time might prove a more sensible starting schedule. It's far easier to succeed and increase your workouts, than to overdo it, fail and have to regroup.

Perhaps your situation is different. Perhaps you're used to being in excellent shape and working out regularly. But something has come up—a new baby, a company merger—and you've let your exercising slide by the wayside for several months. One day you try to zip up your pants, and guess what? The zipper won't close.

So you decide to get back into the exercise groove. Good. You were used to running five miles a day, so that's what you decide to do. Uh oh. Bad.

Start slow. Give yourself a chance to work back into shape. Don't get discouraged. Your body knows what to do—your muscle memory will speed up along the path to fitness—and it will respond.

Quitting is so easy. If you're looking for a reason to quit, you surely will: you're busy at work, the gym's too far away, your shoes are losing their cushioning, on and on. Odds are nobody is going to rise and give a blood oath to stand by you as you exercise, through thick and thin. Odds are nobody's going to care all that much—at least not enough to convince you to exercise—and certainly not as much as you should care.

Keep it sane and simple.

2 **Do what you can to prevent injuries.** It is vital to know when to pause and rest. It does no good to work yourself into terrific shape by running long distances only to ignore warning pain and break your body down in the process. Listen to your body; when it tells you to take a break, take a break. That break will allow you to come back even stronger.

For many, it's so hard to stop exercising, even for a day, no matter what the aches and pains. Exercising becomes addictive. The feeling of your blood racing through your arteries and veins, working and building your muscles, can produce a unique high.

Even so, you must use your common sense. Stop when your body tells you to, no matter how hard it is to pull away from the treadmill or weight bench.

Another aspect of preventing injuries has to do with equipment. First and foremost, that means wearing shoes that fit, are comfortable and designed for the activity you are undertaking. If you're about to start running, make sure you are wearing dependable running shoes. Note: While cross training is great, cross training shoes are not appropriate for every activity, and certainly not for running. You don't need a lot of gear to run, but running shoes absolutely top the list.

3 **Treat an injury intelligently and quickly.** Even when you do everything right, injuries still occur. More often than not, ignoring an injury in typical tough-jock fashion only gives it an opportunity to get worse. If it seems like a minor swelling or pain, use the RICE method:

R   **Rest** the aggrieved area.

I   **Ice** the area for twenty-minute sessions anywhere from 24 to 48 hours after the injury occurs.

C   Apply **compression** or pressure, assuming the injury demands this sort of attention.

E   **Elevate** the area above the heart to reduce swelling.

Don't stop there. Take ibuprofen or another anti-inflammatory drug. Carefully stretch the muscles in the area of the injury.

If all this fails, don't hesitate to call a doctor. A minor injury can become major before you know it.

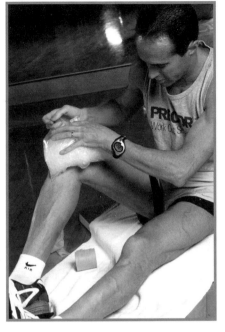

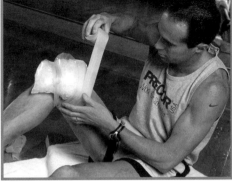

Alberto demonstrates proper ice pack application techniques on his knee.

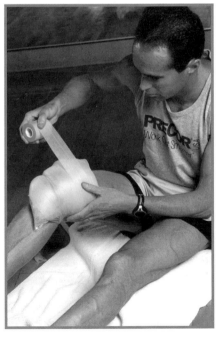

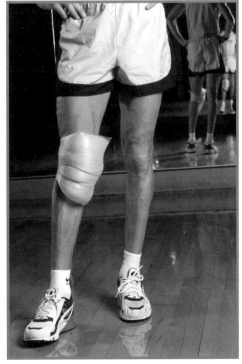

4 **Drink plenty of water or other fluids.** You've most likely heard this often: stay hydrated. Running and other exercises deplete the body of large amounts of fluids, which need to be replaced. If you don't keep yourself hydrated, you leave yourself open to problems that range from muscle cramps, headaches and fatigue to dehydration, which not only is unpleasant but potentially dangerous, even life-threatening. Nothing beats plain old water for most people and events, but if you're running for more than one hour, consider consuming some sports drink

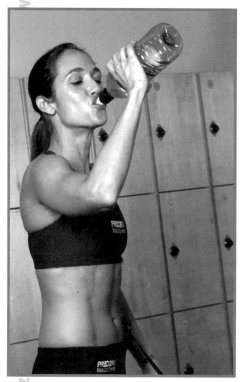

that contains electrolytes. In general, consume one to two cups of fluid before beginning to exercise and then four to eight ounces every 15 minutes during your workout. After your workout, drink two cups of fluid for every pound of body weight lost. Avoid caffeine and alcohol, which as diuretics, will only increase your dehydration.

5 **Stretch.** Many people find it just too hard to bother to stretch, and it's not difficult to understand why. Stretching hardly ranks up there with exciting activities, since the emphasis is on deliberation and precision and getting ready to do something exciting or fun. Nor does stretching give an aerobic high, or pumped up muscles, or any of the usual expressions of immediate gratification. In addition, nobody really seems to know how much stretching is necessary. Should you do it before you run or after—or both? One minute or five or fifteen? Standing up or lying on your back? Good questions, though we'll table these for a moment. The issue of flexibility and stretching is sufficiently important to deserve a separate chapter, and so we'll address this issue in the very next chapter.

Putting that aside, we now hope you recognize the importance of doing whatever you can—from reading to thinking to learning to preparing—to protect your body from the strains and stresses of exercise. After all, the essence of getting fitter is the continual breakdown of the muscles followed by a rebuilding process that renders them stronger—and that's not necessarily a painless process.

That doesn't mean exercise has to be painful—but painless is another matter entirely.

On to stretching . . .

CHAPTER 3

Stretching and Flexibility

STRETCHING HAS COME A LONG WAY in the past few years. It used to be the unloved stepchild of a typical exercise program. Some people did it, some avoided it, but few claimed to enjoy it, and precious few were interested in talking about it.

Those were the old days. Things have changed, at least as far as the acknowledged importance of stretching is concerned. The American College of Sports Medicine recently released new guidelines that rank flexibility—defined as the range of motion around a joint—along with cardiovascular conditioning and muscular strength a major component of fitness. While athletes always have recognized the importance of stretching to increase flexibility, this new appreciation is beginning to reach the general population, helped along by doctors, physical therapists and personal trainers.

This change in perception is due to several factors. The demographically crucial baby boomer generation is aging—more than 80 million Americans are at least 35 years old—and finding itself increasingly beset by common physical ailments, such as bad backs, stiffness, arthritis. All of us, whether baby boomer or not, face two competing realities: we wish to remain physically functional throughout our increasingly long lives, yet at the same time we are the least active, most machine-dependent human beings ever to have walked (or sat) on this planet. Few of us hunt for our own food, build our own homes, plant our own gardens, or hike to work. In fact, we spend a disproportionate amount of our days hunching in front of a computer monitor, sitting behind the wheel, talking on the phone or lying comatose in front of the television.

In the old days, we were constantly on the move, as a matter of self-preservation. While no one—no one reasonably sane, that is—would advocate a return to hustling on a daily basis for survival, our modern sedentary existence can be as deadly as wrestling with T-Rex over leftovers.

We take it for granted that we will stiffen and become creaky with age. We expect that our joints will hurt, our knees will ache, our backs will throb and there is nothing we can do about it. We know that doctors tell us that most adults over age 30 lose ten percent of their flexibility with each passing decade.

While true for most, it doesn't have to be that way. Given good health, we can be virtually as flexible in our eighties as we are in our twenties. The secret is to remain physically active throughout our lifetimes and incorporate stretching into our lives. Stretching helps lengthen muscle tissues, making them less prone to trauma and tears. It increases flexibility, decreasing the chance of muscle injury and helping to maintain function.

In addition to preventing injury and maintaining function, stretching maximizes performance. To gain the most from your physical activity, you must employ each muscle's capacity to the utmost. The looser you are from stretching, the easier it will be to progress through a wider range of motion, and the less energy it will cost you to complete the motion.

Examples from the running world: If your hamstrings are very tight, your stride length will be limited because your knees won't be able to swing as high and as forward as they should be able to. This will cause you to travel less distance through the air with each stride. Likewise, if your quadriceps are suffering from the same tightness as your hamstrings, your "push-off" leg (the leg that is propelling you forward and off the earth) will be pulled off the ground prematurely, before you achieve maximum extension and force, thereby shortening each stride and depriving you of the ability to move forward as fast and as far as you could.

Now that we have established that stretching counts, in so many ways, what do we do about it?

Stretching Basics

We all learned a few stretches in school: down on your back, leg crooked at the knee, pushing away from the body; standing up, angled against a wall, elbows bent, feet flat on the ground; arms behind the back, one hand grasping the wrist of the other, pulling.

Stretching also involves warming up before you exercise and cooling down afterwards. Warm ups and cool downs are essential segments of your workout session and normally should involve lighter intensity versions of your workout. For instance, you might walk or jog slowly for five to 10 minutes before running. Or, you might start out by running slowly and easily before gaining some speed to stretch your muscles and prepare your body for the challenge ahead.

When holding traditional stretches, it is essential to focus on individual muscle groups in your legs—quadriceps, hamstrings, shins and calves, as well as the muscles in your shoulders and arms. Done properly, a few minutes a day is all it takes for most people to gain the benefit they seek and need from stretching.

Each movement should be smooth and steady. Never bounce in a stretch or make quick, abrupt movements. Never stretch to the point of causing pain. And make sure you do long static stretching (holding the stretches without bouncing) at the end of your workout. Research has shown that stretching after your cool down, when your muscles are still warm, can be more important than stretching before your workout.

Since most people don't have a lot of time to devote to stretching, concentrate on the major muscle groups to stay flexible. If you are so inclined, find out about stretching exercises that reach the smaller muscles as well, and give them a try. The effort surely won't be wasted, for, as the song goes, ". . . the foot bone's connected to the ankle bone, the ankle bone's connected to the shin bone . . ." Think of the body as one, big link; the more flexible the individual parts, the more flexible the entire mechanism.

Serious and professional athletes have to approach stretching differently. Most begin with 10 to 15 minutes of some light activity, such as jogging, biking, or jumping rope. Once they build up to a sweat and their muscles are feeling warm, they stretch for five to 10 minutes before beginning their primary exercise or activity. Once they finish their workout, they ordinarily stretch for 10 to 15 minutes to maintain their flexibility, in preparation for the next training session.

Right there, you can see one example of the differences between serious athletes and people who are simply trying to get into reasonable shape. Those in the latter group might spend a total of 30 minutes a day exercising, while serious athletes could easily spend at least half that time just stretching. Therefore, while it is imperative for everyone to stretch, the less serious athletes can only afford to spend a few minutes out of their relatively short exercise session doing so. Those few minutes must be put to use in the most efficient manner possible.

Sample Stretches

In order to assist you in achieving maximum efficiency, Isabel Lorca is on hand to provide her stretching routine. It would be hard to find anyone better positioned to offer this sort of advice.

Isabel was a classically trained dancer, an accomplished actor, and a competitive triathlete when she survived a severe car accident in 1992. Another vehicle ran a red light and smashed into her car, causing her to

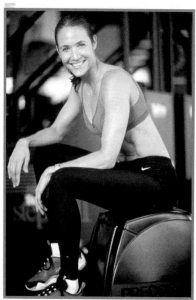

Isabel Lorca

fly through the windshield. Upon landing in the street, she was struck by yet another auto. The crash resulted in serious damage to her spinal cord. Her synapses weren't firing in proper sequence, which meant the signals weren't getting to her brain, telling her how to stand and walk and other fundamentally important things. In addition to this paralysis (which doctors could only hope was temporary), she suffered torn ligaments and broken bones.

After being laid up in bed for nine months, Isabel slowly began to regain her ability to move about on her own. It would take three and half years of hard work before she would regain most of her strength, flexibility and conditioning.

Isabel hadn't only changed physically—she was a different person inside as well. She did not return to her old life and career. Instead, she embarked on a new path, adding a master's degree in sports psychology from U.C.L.A. to go with her B.S. in kinesiology from the College Francais. She became certified in a variety of athletic disciplines by the International Sports Science Association and other certifying organizations, quickly establishing herself as a top trainer in Los Angeles, with movie stars and professional athletes for clients. She also has developed, in conjunction with Precor, a new program for the EFX Elliptical Fitness Crosstrainer.

Isabel generously has provided the following stretching routine that will leave you as limber as can be. Each of the stretches should be held for approximately one minute.

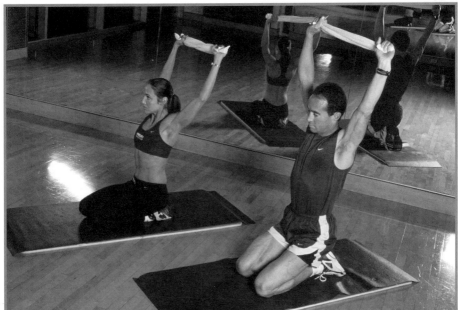

1 Shoulder Joint Flexibility: Hold a stick or towel in both hands, as wide apart as is comfortable. Slowly raise the stick or towel over your head until it is behind you. As your shoulder flexibility improves, you will be able to perform this movement with your hands positioned closer and closer together.

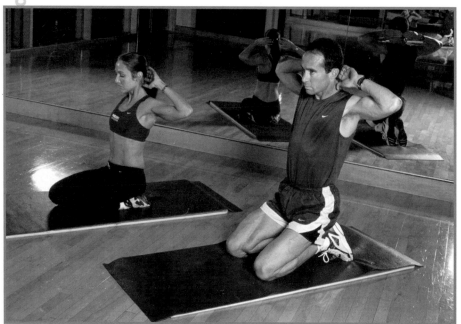

2 **Chest Stretch:** Place your hands behind your head – fingertips touching, elbows out to the side. Slowly press your elbows out behind your body and hold that position. Tilt slightly to the left and hold; tilt slightly to the right and hold.

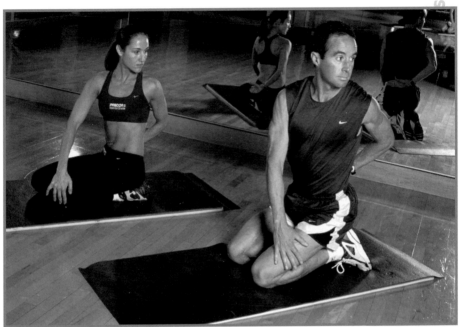

3 **Torso Twists:** Straddle a bench or sit on a mat and hold yourself locked into a seated position. Slowly twist left and then right, over and over, as far as you can reach each time. This twisting motion is terrific for the lower back, but be careful—doing it too fast can be dangerous.

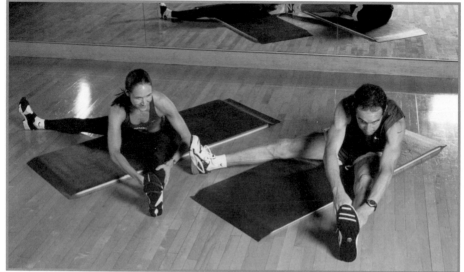

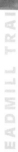

4 Hamstring Stretch: Too many athletes ignore the importance of hamstring flexibility—but you won't. Sit on the floor with your legs spread apart, and lower your chest toward your right leg until you feel tension, then try placing it against your left leg. Finally, push your chest between your legs, straight down toward the ground. This will not only lengthen your hamstrings, it also will improve your hip joint flexibility.

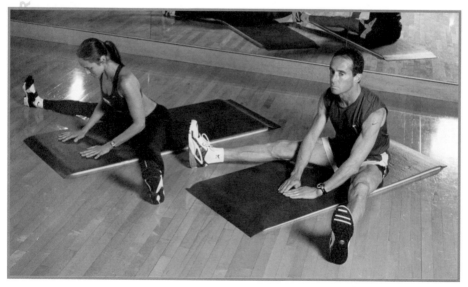

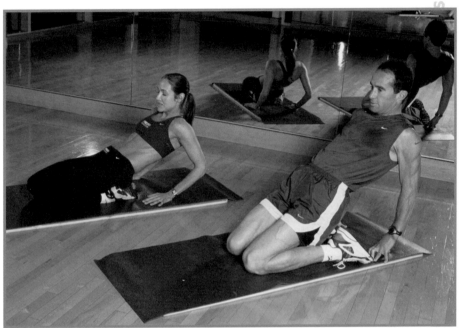

5 **Quadriceps Stretch:** Kneel down and place your hands on the ground behind you. Slowly lean back by sliding your hands backward. You will feel the stretch as you lean back. Hold the position for one minute, remembering to "relax" in the stretch posture.

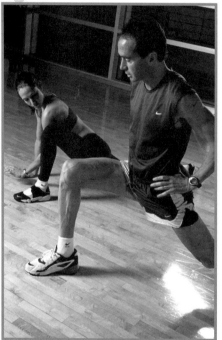 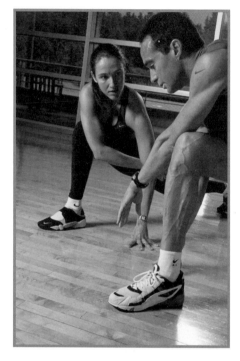

6 **Front Straddle Stretch:** This lunging stretch can be performed either while standing still or walking forward. Stand up straight, head up, back firm, and place your hands on either sides of your right leg or on your hips. Move that leg forward until your knee is bent (at approximately a 90-degree angle) directly over your foot. Keeping your head and back straight, lower your body as close to the ground as possible, and hold the position. Switch legs and repeat. Again, you can do this stretch standing still, bringing your leg back and remaining in one spot, or you can slowly walk forward while lunging.

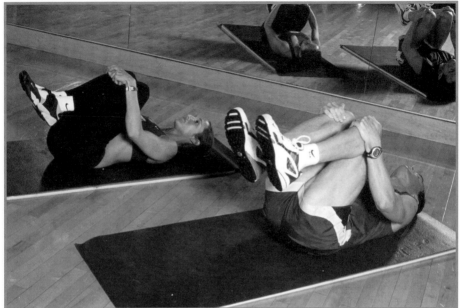

7 Lower Back Stretch: Lay on the floor on your back, with your knees bent. Gently pull both knees toward your chest, lifting your feet off the floor. Hold and relax. As an alternative, you can perform this concentrating on one leg at a time.

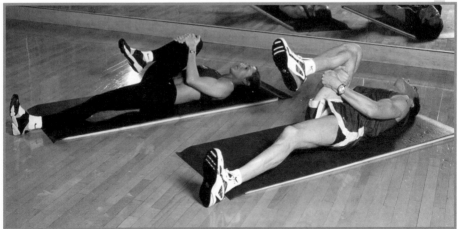

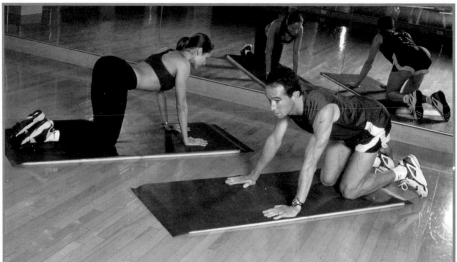

8 **Cat Stretch (also stretches lower back):** Get on your hands and knees, and let your back sag while lifting your head up. Round your back, and lower your chin to your chest. Hold for several seconds, and then repeat.

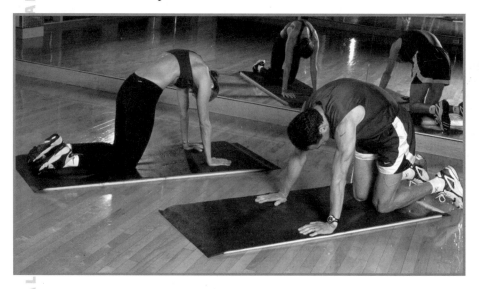

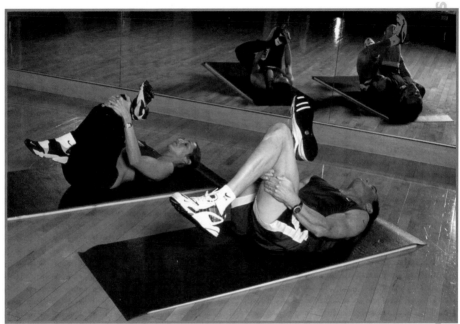

9 **Outer Hip Stretch:** You're back on your back for this one. In
that position, flex your right knee across your body and press it
down toward your left shoulder. Repeat on the other side.

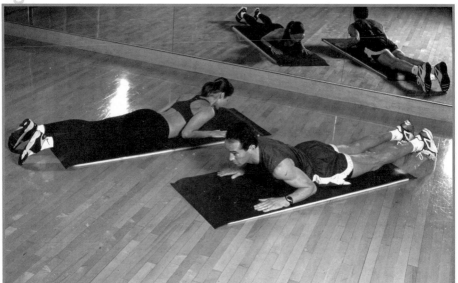

10 **Torso Stretch:** Lay on your stomach with your hands in the push-up position (palms flat on the floor straight down from your shoulders.) Slowly lift your upper body, keeping your hips and lower body on the floor. As an easier alternative, you can perform this stretch keeping your forearms on the ground. Be sure to do this within a pain-free range only, which of course is true for all stretches.

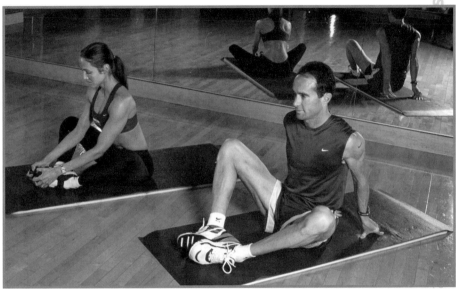

11 **Groin Stretch:** Sit erect on the floor, with the soles of your feet together, legs straight out. Gently pull your heels towards your groin. Press the inside of your knees towards the floor. Hold the stretch.

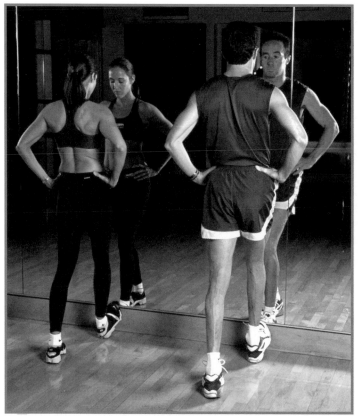

Standing Calf Stretch

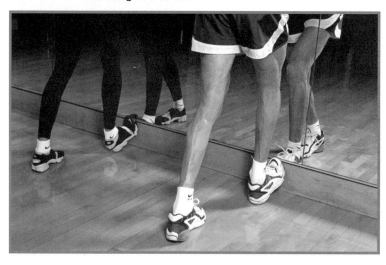

12 Calf Stretch: This one is divided into two parts because changing the angle of the knee accentuates different calf muscles.

Standing Calf Stretch: Stand facing a wall and place one foot behind the other. With your front knee slightly bent, your back knee straight and your heel down, press your toes against the wall. Repeat on the opposite side.

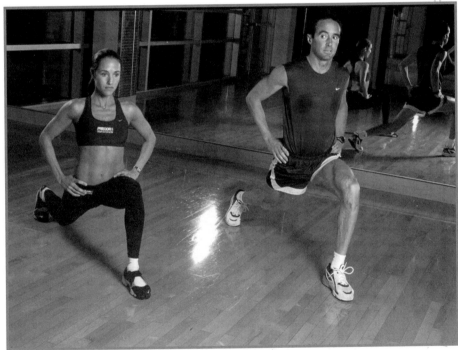

Achilles Stretch

Achilles Stretch: With your hands on your hips, place one foot behind the other. With both your knees bent, lean forward from the hips, feeling the stretch in your Achilles tendon. Repeat on the opposite side.

A caveat: It is crucial to remember that while all these are legitimate and effective stretches, they are imprecise. Pull too far or push too hard or don't hold it long enough, and you won't be getting the maximum benefit from your stretch. Stretching is not like lifting weights or running five miles, where the measures are fairly absolute. Stretching is a matter of feel and adjustment, of awareness and control, of sensitivity and responsiveness, those things at which most of us are not very good.

In response, some manufacturers are beginning to seek a technological solution to human imprecision. In fact, Precor has devised the Precor Stretch Trainer, which effectively stretches all major muscle groups without risk of injury or discomfort. Dr. James Crivello, chiropractor and the inventor of the Stretch Trainer, licensed his breakthrough machine to Precor. Numerous studies have been conducted to document its effectiveness. According to *Fitness Industry Technology*, biomechanical research undertaken at the University of Oregon by Dr. Barry Bates demonstrated that the Stretch Trainer "enhanced back and hamstring flexibility over an extended period." Other studies documented an improvement in coordination and power transfer, and confirmed that the unit was more effective than simply stretching on the floor.

Stretch Safely

Here are some things to keep in mind when you stretch to ensure that your routine is as safe and effective as possible:

- Stretch both before and after your activity.
- Stretch daily.
- Move slowly into each stretch, never use jarring motion.
- Breathe deeply as you hold each stretch, without bouncing, for at least 15 seconds* (the longer the better).
- Ease up on the stretch if your muscles start to shake.
- Never stretch to the point of pain—you should feel only tension in the muscles, which should dissipate, as you hold your stretch.

*Results of a recent study published in the *British Medical Journal* suggest that while holding a stretch at least 15 seconds is optimal, five or 10 seconds will still improve your range of motion. Just do it!

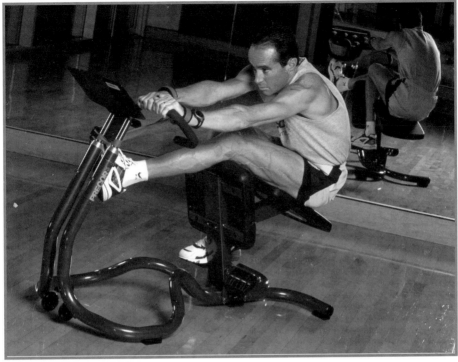

The Stretch Trainer is so effective and safe because, unlike traditional stretching, the machine uses the body's own weight to achieve a full stretch. The individual stays securely seated throughout the exercises, which stabilizes the back, and keeps the pelvis and knees in place. This security and stability reduces the chance of pain or injury. Furthermore, the individual remains in complete control of each stretch by gently rocking backwards in the pivot seat, holding on to the handlebar. All shifts into new stretches are performed from a static position, eliminating the possibility of slipping or unexpectedly moving in a way that could cause injury.

A complete session takes about eight to 10 minutes, and should be done four times a week. Whether you stretch on the ground or with a machine, stretching is vital to any successful exercise program.

Now that you are properly stretched, and well on the path to preserving and even increasing your flexibility, let's get on the treadmill. It's time to walk, cross train, and run, run, run.

TRAINING AND WORKOUT GUIDE

CHAPTER 4
Walk Your Way to Fitness

HUMAN BEINGS ARE PRETTY GOOD AT WALKING. Most of learn to walk before we learn to speak. In fact, most of learn to walk before we learn to do much of anything.

By this time, you are undoubtedly adept at walking. So let's put your considerable skill to good use.

Fundamentally, walking and running are similar. One primary difference is that, given equal conditions, the heart rate increases more during running than when walking normally (as distinguished from racewalking, which can raise the heart rate to running levels). At the same time, there is considerably less pounding—approximately half, for the average person—endured by your body when walking, because your legs don't travel as far, as fast or as high as they do when running. Since each running step lands with the equivalent of three to five times your body weight (the variance due to individual physiology and movement), we're talking about real stress on your joints, bones, etc.

So while you may not work quite as hard walking, you won't suffer the same strains, either. The first half of that equation can be altered, and the effort expended while walking dramatically increased, by raising the grade on your treadmill, so you are walking uphill. The steeper the incline, the more strenuous the walk, and the harder your heart works.

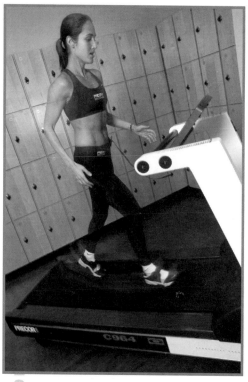

ALBERTO SALAZAR: THE TREAD

So let's get something clear right at the start — walking isn't a poor substitute for running, the easy way out for those not tough enough to get up and sprint around the track until blinded by sweat and hobbled by cramps. In 1994, one of the co-authors of this book, Alberto Salazar was only two months away from competing in the Olympic Trials Marathon when he sustained a stress fracture in his foot, which led to a tremendous dilemma. Alberto couldn't afford to simply sit in his chaise lounge and wait six weeks for the injury to heal, so he maintained his extraordinarily high level of fitness by walking uphill on a treadmill with a 15 percent grade.

Walking uphill raised Alberto's heart rate much higher than if he had jogged on flat ground at a nine-minute pace, which would not only have proved despairingly slow, (at least for Alberto), but also would have aggravated his foot. After sticking to this uphill walking routine through the course of his injury, Alberto was able to return to running, gradually increase his mileage, and make the Olympic team.

Many surgeries later, Alberto remains a believer. He still walks uphill on a treadmill to recover after each medical intervention, sometimes wearing a weighted vest to increase the difficulty. Once he is able to resume running, he finds that it only take about two weeks to get his "running legs" back, thanks to the walking.

If it works for our co-author, imagine the benefits the less serious athlete can accrue. At a reasonable minimum, which would mean a half-hour exercise session — an amount of time doctors commonly recommend for raising your heart rate— done about four times a week, you will achieve substantial aerobic benefits.

Walking Is Good For Body And Brain

In case you need more encouragement to get out and walk, a study reported in the journal *Nature* points to another significant benefit of walking. Researchers at the University of Illinois recruited 124 sedentary volunteers aged 60 to 75 and assigned different exercises: half were given an anaerobic program, which incorporated stretching and weight lifting, and the other half were given a walking program. The study was six months in duration, and the walkers were eventually able to complete an hour-long loop around the university campus, three times a week. Because the participants were not exercisers before joining the study, it was relatively easy to measure the difference that exercise did or did not make. The results were quite intriguing.

It turned out that walking provided not only a good workout for the body, but also for the brain. Both memory and judgment were sharpened in the walking group. Brain functions known as "executive control processes," which are located in the brain's frontal and prefrontal lobes, and include the ability to plan, set schedules, make a choice, remember that choice, and quickly change that choice were enhanced in the walkers. Executive control is essential to our ability to be independent, to live on our own.

It's never too late. Whether you are 75 or 25, walking can do so much for you, and that means for all of you, body and brain.

"These areas of the brain decline the earliest with aging," explains Dr. Arthur Kramer, a cognitive neuroscientist, and the study's lead author, in a *New York Times* article. "So executive control is more severely affected by the normal aging process than other brain functions."

The study employed simple chores to gauge the participants' level of executive control. For instance, in an exercise known as "task switching," the volunteers were shown alternating letters and numbers, and asked to instantly distinguish between vowels and consonants, and between odd and even numbers. The walkers improved their task switching capability by 25 percent. At the same time, those who lifted weights and stretched did not find their competence in this area enhanced.

Why walking can improve our memory and planning abilities, and perhaps even our general mental acuity is uncertain, but the encouraging results are undeniable. And they offer the promise of a happier life for all, no matter where they now stand on the fitness scale. To quote Dr. Kramer once more:

> "People who have chosen a lifetime of inactivity can benefit mentally from improved aerobic fitness. It's never too late."

Remember those words: *It's never too late.* Whether you are 75 or 25, walking can do so much for you, and that means for all of you, body and brain.

Walking Is Great For Pregnant Women

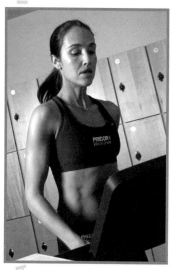

We have yet to mention a vitally important category of walkers: pregnant women. Doctors increasingly recognize the importance of staying in shape during pregnancy, and many women, who already jog or run, continue to do so after they conceive. In fact, some women runners keep running right through their pregnancy, literally to the day of delivery. This latter group does not constitute the majority, and are usually very strong, fit runners.

At the same time, starting a running program while pregnant is not a good idea, nor is pushing your body too far. Raising your body temperature too high (above 100.4 degrees F) can damage the fetus. Of course you should consult your physician to determine the proper exercise program for you.

Having said that, walking is a terrific exercise for pregnant women. The basic goal of running is to keep your pulse rate up so that you are conditioning your heart and gaining cardiovascular fitness as well as burning calories. Walking can accomplish that too, without the pounding and bouncing, which can only be that much more uncomfortable during pregnancy. Walking will elevate your heart rate, and you won't have to worry about the injuries or over-exertion associated with running. Please note that the American College of Gynecologists and Obstetricians' guidelines recommend that pregnant women should modify exercise intensity according to how they feel and should stop exercising when they feel fatigued. Women may find that their training heart rates during pregnancy need to be lower than their pre-pregnancy rates.

Walking Programs

Now that you know the benefits of walking, here is an exercise routine brought to us by Paul Frediani, a personal trainer, athlete and author from New York. You'll hear more from Paul in the next chapter, but right now, the following is his contribution to walking on the treadmill. He calls the program the Mountain Climber.

The Mountain Climber

The Mountain Climber is a simple and terrific cardio walking workout, that provides much of the benefits of running without the pounding. It involves walking intervals of varying grades.

1 Warm up for 5 minutes by walking, starting slowly and gradually increasing your speed until you reach your brisk fitness walking pace. Your goal is to maintain this brisk pace even as we alter the angle of the treadmill.

2 Walk briskly for 1 minute, setting the treadmill to Level One.

3 Raise the treadmill to Level Two, and walk for 1 minute.

4 Return to Level One for 1 minute.

5 Raise to Level Three for 1 minute.

6 Return to Level One for 1 minute.

7 Raise to Level Four for 1 minute.

8 Return to Level One for 1 minute.

9 Raise to Level Five for 1 minute.

10 Return to Level One for 1 minute.

11 Cool down for 5 minutes, gradually reducing your speed.

Obviously, you can raise the grade higher as you become more fit, as well as increase your walking pace, and the duration of each stage. This exercise is a terrific use of the treadmill, taking advantage of the machine's attributes that allow you to work you legs and heart safely, in different ways.

Climb/Descend

This walking workout consists of a continuous climb, followed by a descent. Try to maintain your workout speed even as the incline gets steeper.

1 Warm up for 5 minutes by walking at Level One, gradually increasing your speed to the desired workout pace.

2 Walk briskly at Level One for 2 minutes.

3 Raise to Level Two for 2 minutes.

4 Raise to Level Three for 2 minutes.

5 Raise to Level Four for 2 minutes.

6 Raise to Level Five for 4 minutes.

7 Lower to Level Four for 2 minutes.

8 Lower to Level Three for 2 minutes.

9 Lower to Level Two for 2 minutes.

10 Lower to Level One for 2 minutes.

11 Cool down for 5 minutes, gradually reducing speed.

The Plateau Workout

This workout involves a slight climb, followed by a long stretch at the same level, and then a descent. Bear in mind that the levels and durations here are suggestions; just as with your speed, work at levels and for an amount of time that is doable yet challenging.

1 Warm up for 5 minutes by walking at Level One, gradually increasing your speed to the desired workout pace.

2 Walk briskly at Level One for 1 minute.

3 Raise to Level Two for 1 minute.

4 Raise to Level Three (your plateau) for 15–20 minutes.

5 Lower to Level Two for 1 minute.

6 Lower to Level One for 1 minute.

7 Cool down for 5 minutes, gradually reducing your speed.

Racewalking

Finally, let's take a moment to contemplate what you can legitimately regard as the ultimate in walking: racewalking. Racewalking might look strange, but it's fantastic exercise, without running's tremendous pounding on your limbs and joints — and if you get good enough, you can make it to the Olympics on Team USA.

Racewalking is not simply walking really fast. In fact, it occupies that space and velocity between walking and running, where you are moving too fast to normally walk, and you're ready to break into a run but you don't. Instead, you racewalk.

To begin, one foot must always maintain contact with the ground, with the leg straight. This fundamental rule accounts for the funny wobbling motion that we see in racewalkers.

To racewalk, the heel should strike the ground, and the toes should be facing skyward. The step is united into a continuous motion, as one foot rolls forward, in perfect opposition to the other foot, which is landing on its heel. Unlike running, in which the athlete gets to float through the air for an instant before touching ground, racewalkers never get that break because their feet are always in contact with the ground. That forces them to constantly tighten, flex and therefore work their muscles. That is neither easy nor effortless. That is working hard.

Simultaneously, the arms should swing in a tight arc, the thumbs traveling from the waist to the chest, crooked into an L shape. The arms swing as fast as the legs. Your hips should swivel not so much side to side, but rather front to back, assisting the arms and legs to stay in control and in rapid motion.

Doing all this correctly requires you to contract the muscles in your stomach and your butt, providing each area with a rigorous workout.

The accomplished racewalker reaps the benefits from his efforts: he not only will strengthen his shins, calves, glutes and abs, but will burn more calories than a runner, assuming they travel at similar speeds. Racewalking at 5.5 miles per hour is just as hard a workout as running at 6.5 MPH.

A number of coaches, clinics and associations, including The North American Racewalking Foundation, can help you to learn to racewalk properly. They can be located easily in the phone book or on the web.

Despite racewalking's many benefits, it has long suffered from an image problem. After all, it does look kind of funny, especially when you're not all that experienced and polished at it, and this has caused many people to shy away from racewalking.

But that's the beauty of the treadmill. You're not out on that big, broad public street, you're safe and secure within the confines of either your home or gym, working away on your favorite treadmill. Keep the world out, and racewalk — swivel and swagger — to your heart's content.

CHAPTER 5
Cross Training

NIKKI STONE WAS ALMOST WHERE SHE WANTED TO BE, which was on top of her game. She had spent a majority of her 24 years learning to ski, practicing and perfecting her technique, and competing. All that work, combined with her talent, had paid off: Nikki was ranked second in the world in freestyle aerial skiing, a difficult, demanding sport where creativity, daring and athleticism are paramount.

Now Nikki stood on a peak in Europe, in the midst of another competition on the women's skiing tour. The number one skier had stumbled in her last turn, and Nikki saw the chance to move ahead and take the top spot. All she had to do was to hit her next run just right.

But Nikki wasn't feeling quite right. Her back was hurting badly and she wondered whether it was smart to ski any more that day. Her competitive fire overruled her hesitancy, and off she went, bound for glory.

As soon as she lifted off, flying 50 feet

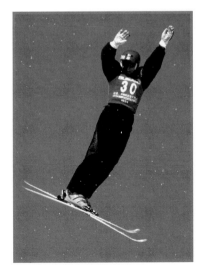

Nikki Stone

into the air, Nikki knew she was in trouble. Her back had given out, and she lost the ability to move it in any familiar pattern. The landing was a rude return to earth, a horribly agonizing smack. Nikki had to be helped off the course, and would have to stay in bed for several days before the pain subsided enough for her to board a plane back to the United States.

Once home, the doctors delivered some bad news. She had severely compressed her spine. In addition, she suffered an anterior tear and fluid was leaking out of her spinal column.

Explaining the damage in simplest terms, the doctors said the injury was analogous to an egg that had been vigorously shaken: the outside looked okay, but the inside was a mess.

Surgery was the only course open to her, and it hardly promised a full recovery. Not only was Nikki out for the season, and the next Olympics, she could forget about skiing ever again, competitively or otherwise.

The prognosis was unacceptable to Nikki. She refused to allow her career to be derailed—not without a fight. She decided against surgery. Despite the warnings from her doctors, she resolved to work herself back into shape, to recover on her own terms, to get strong, ski and compete again, come what may.

In spite of the serious nature of her injury, Nikki had one advantage. She started off in tremendous physical condition, her 5 foot 7 inch frame packed with approximately 130 pounds of lean muscle. Just as important, her determination was fierce.

She set to work, aided by a cadre of physicians and trainers, on a cross training program. She began by walking on the treadmill, working up to one hour a day, a couple of times a week. With time, she started to walk faster, and eventually began running. Even though freestyle skiing demanded short bursts of intense energy rather than the stamina required of endurance sports, Nikki always liked running, which helped her stick to her training.

However, she recognized that she could overdo the running, which would prove too stressful for her back, so she climbed aboard the Precor EFX Elliptical Fitness Crosstrainer four or five times a week, working up to an hour a session. The EFX provided her with the low impact aerobic workouts she needed, which reduced the possibility of straining her joints. A prime advantage to using the EFX was that it was so easy on her back that she began to ski and jump again. (The EFX will be discussed in some depth a bit later in this chapter.)

Nikki also spent many hours lifting weights, especially concentrating on strengthening the muscles that supported her back and legs.

Through her determination, effort and perseverance, Nikki was able to return to the sport she loved. Her goal was absolute, as was her timetable, and she kept to both to the end. Two years after she was hurt on the mountain and told she probably never would ski again, Nikki Stone won the Olympic gold meal in freestyle aerial skiing.

Of course, not everyone has the time, physical ability, or pure will to rehabilitate in the manner that Nikki did. After all, if you're not a world-class skier in the first place, getting injured is not the recommended route to becoming one.

The point is that no one exercise, neither skiing nor treadmill running, provided the total answer for Nikki. Likewise, while running promises a fantastic workout, spicing up your exercise sessions with some other types of activities can only help you meet or exceed your goals.

This doesn't necessarily mean you have to leave the treadmill. In fact, Paul Frediani uses the treadmill to construct an all-around, cross training workout.

Treadmill Cross Training

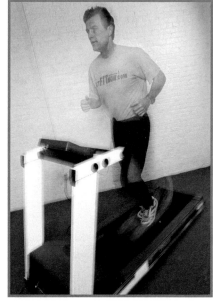

Before we begin discussing cross training on the treadmill, let's not forget the *caveats*: Though the following exercises were developed to take advantage of the treadmill's abilities, the treadmill was built specifically with walking and running in mind. Don't consider attempting any of these exercises without evaluating all safety issues. If you decide to try them, make sure you have a friend or trainer alongside in case of a misstep. Start slowly, cautiously, and very carefully. No manufacturer (or probably any-

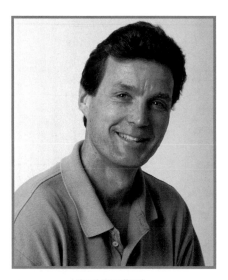

Paul Frediani

body else, for that matter), is going to insure you against injury when you use the equipment in a manner that it has not been expressly designed for, so try these at your own risk.

Having said all that, here are personal trainer Paul Frediani's innovations. You might find them intriguing and worth your time. You might want to give one or more of them a try. The choice is yours.

Paul has an impressively varied resume. A Diamond Belt light heavyweight boxing champion from his hometown in San Francisco, he also won the light heavyweight title in the Golden Gloves in San Francisco. Now a personal trainer in New York, Paul is certified by the American College of Sports Medicine and is a continuing educator provider for the American Council on Exercise. In addition, he is the author of **The Boot Camp Workout** and *Golf Flex: Ten Minutes a Day to Better Play*.

The Lunge

Paul's innovative use of the treadmill helps to strengthen the leg muscles in ways that running does not. A prime example of this is lunging, which is a terrific exercise to build the quadriceps, hamstrings, abdominals, and calves. We discussed lunging in the chapter on stretching, and will describe the form again here. Stand straight while thrusting one leg far out front, so that upon landing, the knee is bent directly over the foot. As a consequence, the entire body follows and has to bend to maintain equilibrium. Continue to keep your head up and back straight. The lunge should be conducted slowly, deliberately and smoothly, without stopping and starting, or any hitches in the action.

Once in this position, repeat the exercise with the other leg, and continue to alternate legs.

Lunging is a strenuous exercise that requires some concentration to ensure that the lunge is performed properly in order to maximize its

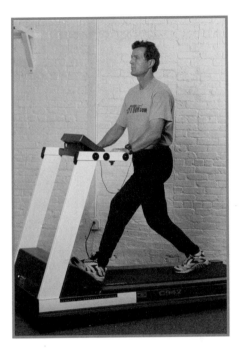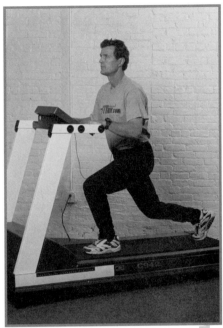

benefits and minimize the risks of imbalance and over-extension. Unfortunately, most people lunge in crowded gyms where they have to wend a winding path, dodging machines and fellow members. Using the treadmill to lunge erases that problem. More importantly, the treadmill's constant motion alters some of the exercise's protocols.

For example, placement of the knee directly over the foot is not a critical factor on the treadmill because the belt's action pushes the leg quickly back to the body, reducing the risk of over-reaching and straining the knee.

Before stepping on the treadmill, practice lunging on solid ground. Then do not hesitate to hold on to the side rails for balance.

Start by setting the machine at .5 to 1.5 MPH, depending on what's comfortable for you. Try 30 seconds of lunging, followed by one minute of walking, and then another 30 seconds of lunging. Do this for a few rounds, though not so long that your form deteriorates and you risk potential injury. Keep going until you can alternate lunging with walking at one-minute intervals, for a total of eight minutes.

Beyond that, you can increase lunging as you see fit. Again, make sure that you don't lunge past your ability to maintain proper form.

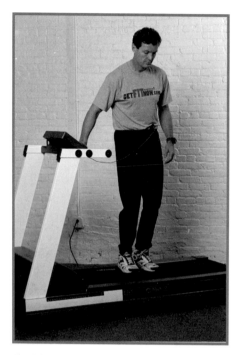

Start by stepping onto the treadmill and turning to the left.

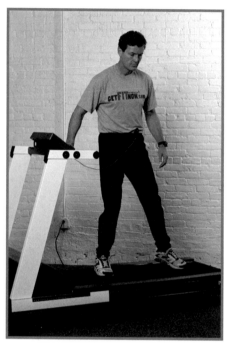

Step sideways with the right leg about shoulder length in width.

Side-stepping

Another one of Paul's special exercises for the treadmill is side-stepping, and its closely related cousin, karaoke. We'll start with side-stepping. You start by stepping onto the treadmill and turning to the left, so your right leg is next to the control panel. Hold on to the rail for balance. Set the treadmill to somewhere between .5 to 1 MPH, depending on what seems right for you.

Step sideways with the right leg—about shoulder length in width, a nice, broad, comfortable step—and then bring the left leg over to meet it. Keep repeating the process, stepping to the side with the right leg and then bringing the left to meet it. This exercise works both the inner thighs and outer thighs, particularly difficult areas to target.

ALBERTO SALAZAR: THE

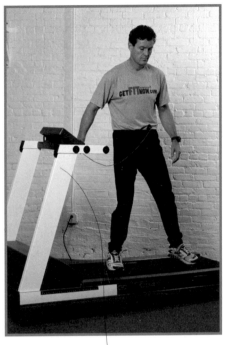

Repeat, stepping to the side with the right leg and bringing the left to meet it.

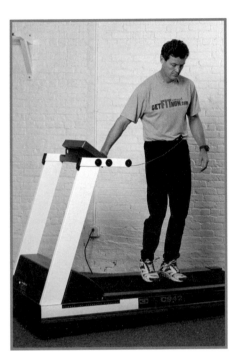

Bring the left leg over to meet the right leg.

Keep side-stepping for one to eight minutes, then stop the machine and turn around, so that your left leg is now next to the control panel. Hold on to the side rail and start side-stepping again. Switching sides allows you to hit all of your thigh muscles.

Karaoke begins the same way. Face the front of the machine, and then turn to the left. Step with the right foot, again about shoulder length in width. However, instead of bringing the left leg over to meet the right, bring the left leg over to cross in front of the right foot. Then the right foot moves back again, stepping out to shoulder length. The left then crosses behind the right leg. Keep going, for as long as you see fit, and then switch sides.

AND WORKOUT GUIDE

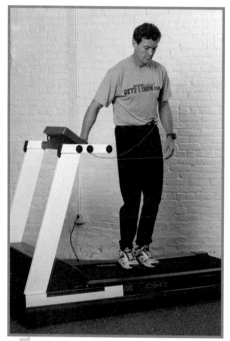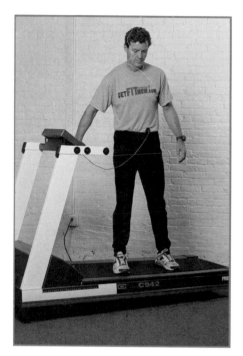

Karaoke Side-stepping

1. Face the front of the treadmill, and then turn to the left.
2. Step with the right foot about shoulder length in width.
3. Bring the left leg over to cross in front of the right foot.
4. Then, the right foot moves back again, stepping out to shoulder length.
5. On the next move, bring your left leg behind your right leg.
6. Finish by returning your legs shoulder width apart.

ALBERTO SALAZAR: THE TREADMILL

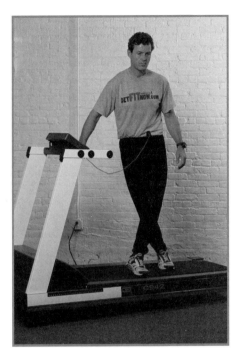
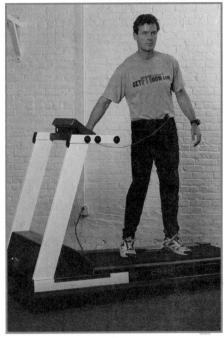
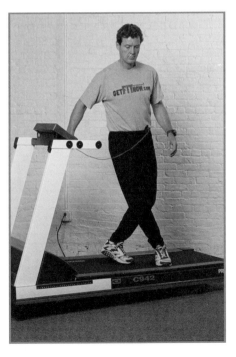
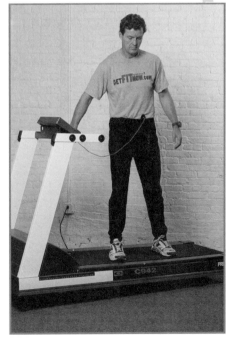

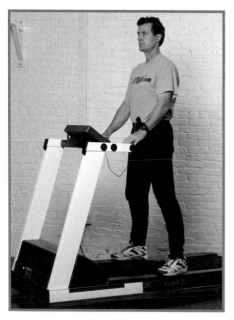

(Above) Stand on the rails of the treadmill, holding onto the bar of the treadmill for balance.

(Below) Bend at the knees 90 degrees, keeping your back straight, head up, chest high, and shoulders back.

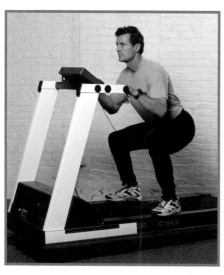

Squats

The squat is an amazing, effective and efficient exercise, providing a complete leg workout from your butt down to your calves. Two variants of the squat—standing and posting—are among Paul's innovative treadmill exercises. Let's quickly explain how to do both of these types of squats, so you can safely perform the exercise.

In the standing squat, stand on the rails of the treadmill. Hold onto the bar if you need to for balance. Bend at the knees, back straight, head up, chest high, shoulders back. Bend to about 90 degrees, keeping the soles of your feet on the rails. When you stand, drive your weight back up through your heels.

The posting modification of the squat adds a tough wrinkle to this classic exercise. Both squats are performed the same way, until you get to the down position with knees flexed at approximately 90 degrees. Before rising from that position, pause to post, as if you were riding a horse (which means lifting up two or three inches, keeping your back straight and your head up, and then returning to your starting position). Post several times when in the down position, and then drive your body all the up, remembering to keep your feet flat on the rails, and to maintain good posture. In addition to all the good that squatting does your lower body, posting gives the gluteals an extra workout.

In one minute you should be able to do a round of 10 standing squats, or 10 posts. A squatting session should consist of three rounds.

Backward Walk

Paul also has incorporated slow backward walking on the treadmill into his exercise regimen. This is mentioned to point out the versatility of the treadmill as an exercise machine. Whatever innovation you think of to help you exercise and achieve the results you seek, may be incorporated into your routine. Always consult a fitness professional or organization such as the American Council on Exercise or American College of Sports Medicine to be sure the movement isn't contraindicated. Also, make sure to add the option cautiously and slowly, increasing intensity, speed and duration only after sufficient practice.

Cross Training Programs

Paul does not use these exercises in isolation. Instead, they are components of entire programs he develops for his clients, designed for people at various stages of fitness, with various interests and goals.

The Butt Burner

For obvious reasons, The Butt Burner is a popular routine. Its specific goal is to tone, shape and define the buttocks.

Begin with 5 minutes of brisk walking, followed by alternating the following exercises in one-minute sessions:

1 Walk briskly at Level One for 2 minutes.

2 Lunge walking.

3 Walking or jogging, (your choice).

4 Standing squats or posting.

5 Walking or jogging.

Repeat this program 5 times.

Cool down for five minutes by walking briskly, then gradually slowing to a stop.

The Leg Toner

Once again begin with 5 minutes of warming up, briskly walking on the treadmill. Then commence with the following exercises, in durations of 1 minute each:

1 Lunge walking.

2 Side-stepping.

3 Backward walking.

4 Karaoke.

Repeat this program 4 times.
End with 5 minutes of walking to cool down.

Other Variations

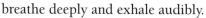

In many ways, these are all variations of a basic theme— get out there and move! Move up, down, even move sideways and backwards. Get your heart rate up and keep it up. Pump your legs and arms. Sweat, breathe deeply and exhale audibly.

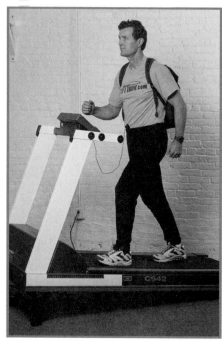

That's it. You've got it. You're there. You're cross training.

In fact, it's a pretty simple recipe for a rather sophisticated-sounding concept.

You might strike upon a variation that suits your specific training needs. For instance, if you're preparing to hike up Mt. Everest, you might want to prepare by angling your treadmill at a steep ascent, and strap on a knapsack loaded with equipment, in order to simulate the conditions you will be experiencing (minus the freezing temperatures, avalanches, white-out emergencies, and other inconveniences.) Note: Of course, while this knapsack innovation provides for a tough, effective workout, if

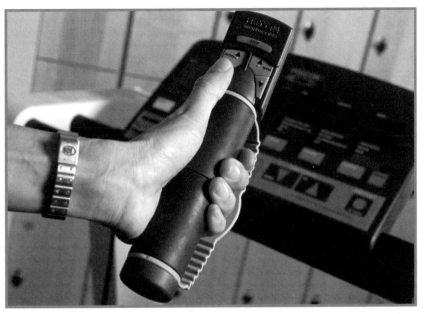

Precor's Smart Weights combine hand weights and a remote control to your treadmill's control panel, allowing you to work the machine without putting down the weights.

you really are planning to take on Everest, this routine alone won't get you to the top. You'll need to do a lot more hard training.

You may also hold weights in your hands as you walk on the treadmill to give your upper body a workout while you're exercising your lower body. While many people find this a valuable training tool, others maintain that carrying extra weight throws off a walker's stride, since your arms cannot swing as freely as when they are unencumbered.

What does seem clear is that if you choose to walk with weights, you should walk, not run. Weights will dramatically, and perhaps dangerously, disrupt your running form, leaving you open to strains and pulls. In addition, carry light weights, one pound or two pounds only, with which you can easily move. Don't forget you're exercising on a constantly moving apparatus, and if you need to suddenly stop or push one of the buttons on the control panel, you'd better be able to react instantly.

Precor manufactures a system of weights with built-in links to the treadmill's control panel, allowing you to work the machine without putting down the weights.

CROSS TRAINING AND WORKOUT GUIDE

The EFX

One of the most valuable weapons in the cross training arsenal is the Precor EFX Elliptical Fitness Crosstrainer. As previously noted, it's the machine Nikki Stone used during her rehabilitation, and it's a machine worth discussing in some detail.

Here's the secret to the elliptical's success: Contrary to the old saying favored by coaches throughout the sports world, the EFX delivers *no pain, all gain.*

Let's talk about the no pain part of the equation first: The Elliptical's motion ranks somewhere between a treadmill, a stairclimber, and a cross-country skier. The feet are placed in pedals, which move neither vertically nor horizontally, but in an oblong fashion, at an angle that varies at the user's discretion, from slightly downhill to flat to far uphill as well

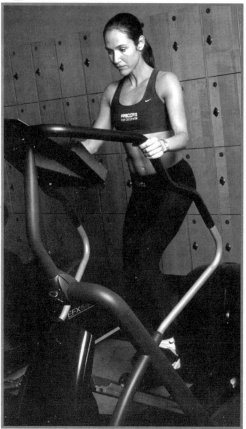

and backward and forward. Because of the oblong motion, the user experiences none of the pounding, bouncing, strain or stress, associated with other cardio machines. To vary the intensity of the workout the resistance can be adjusted at the user's discretion.

There is little doubt that the Elliptical delivers a low-impact workout. But what about the results?

Research conducted at the University of Oregon shows that the Precor EFX exercises the gluteal muscles 30 percent more effectively than steppers, and the quadriceps 60 percent more thoroughly than most cardiovascular machines. Other studies have demonstrated that an elliptical machine provides at least as productive a workout as any type of cardiovascular equipment.

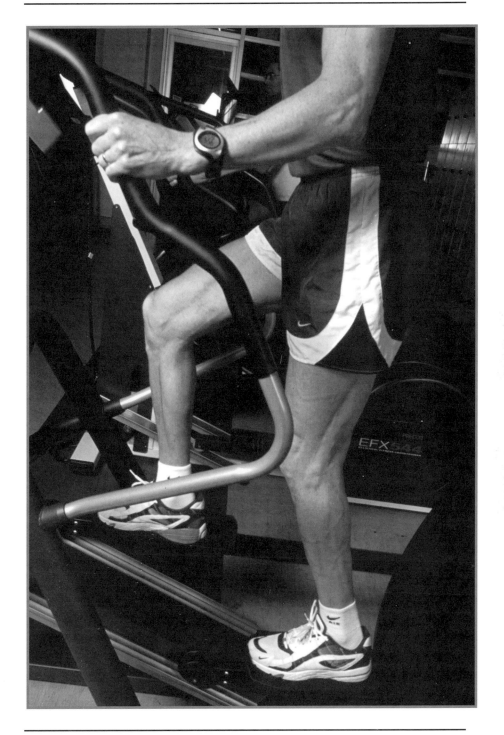

Why Cross Train?

Cross training simply means engaging in a variety of exercises, instead of doing the same routine day in and out. Because this type of training recruits more muscle fibers, as well as works them differently, it stimulates additional strength and overall fitness gains. Other important benefits of cross training include increased compliance to an exercise program, increased motivation (you don't get bored because you're not doing the same thing all the time), and reduced risk of injury because you don't overuse any single muscle group.

What is most interesting is that the rating of perceived exertion (RPE)—a numerical rating of perceived exercise intensity—is lower on the Elliptical than on any other aerobic machine. A study at the University of Mississippi found that subjects experienced more enjoyable workouts, and that their heart rates were higher than they estimated using the RPE scale. The implication is that those using the Elliptical are likely to exercise more frequently and more intensely than those using other machines, because it doesn't *feel* so hard.

So let's add one more vital component to the tally: *No pain, all gain, and more incentive to exercise.*

To reiterate, cross training can include any number of exercises, from running to cycling to swimming, tennis, volleyball, and so on. The virtually infinite range of activities means that while the treadmill can provide you with a variety of exercises that can create an effective cross training routine, you also can step off the treadmill and cross train in a wide range of sports, games, drills and activities. Whatever you decide, make sure you work out consistently and choose activities that target different muscle groups to maximize your benefit.

CHAPTER 6
Running: General Principles

IT'S TIME TO GET TO THE HEART OF THE MATTER: running. After all, most of you are reading this book because you intend to run, and to do that running on the treadmill.

So let's talk about running.

Proper Form

Let's begin with a discussion about form. From beginner to expert, form is of paramount importance. Proper form increases your running efficiency and helps prevent injury. While every person's body, and therefore running motion, is different, there are certain universal fundamentals.

First, maintain an erect posture when running. (Just as your mother told you to do when sitting and walking.) When you lean forward or to the side, you're working against gravity — and gravity always wins. Keep your head, neck, shoulders, spine, hips and legs in line, perpendicular to the ground — and to the force of gravity.

At the same time, it is important to stay relaxed, to keep your body tall and straight without tensing or clenching, and without expending the energy necessary to do that tensing and clenching. Relax your hands

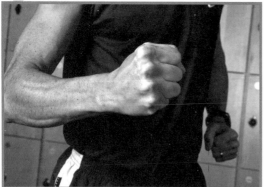

WRONG

Consider gravity again, and let it work for you, as your arms move effortlessly up and down, elbows close to the body, wrists relaxed, hands moving easily up and down, palms facing down, fingers slightly cupped.

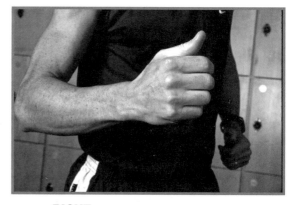

RIGHT

and jaw, and your entire upper body. Let them flow along for the run, as your legs do the work. Consider gravity again, and let it work for you, as your arms move effortlessly up and down, elbows close to the body, wrists relaxed, hands moving easily up and down, palms facing down, fingers slightly cupped.

Land slightly on your heel and midfoot, rapidly shift your weight forward, and push off for the next step. Run lightly, keeping your stride well within your reach, not attempting to stride too far, too long, too wide. Breathe deeply, taking in more oxygen than normal. Fill up your chest with oxygen, which will be that much easier to do because your body will be erect and your chest open. Run forward, which seems obvious, until you stop and observe how many people often run side-to-side especially around their hips.

A word of caution: For all the talk about proper running mechanics, running is an utterly natural act, and you shouldn't try to twist your body into postures it doesn't want to adopt. This is particularly true when it comes to foot placement. While heel-to-toe is the preferred motion for most people, some normally land mid-foot, then briefly rock back on their heels before pushing off on the balls of their feet. (This is true not only for casual runners, but

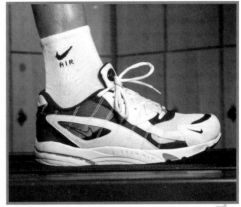

RIGHT

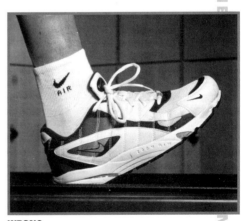

WRONG

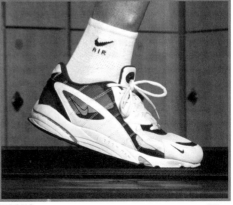

WRONG

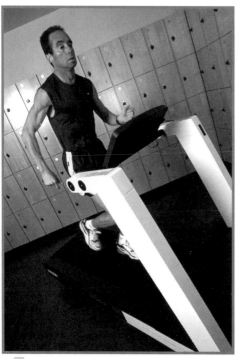

also for some top athletes.) If your body doesn't move naturally a certain way, don't force it. It is possible that by landing on your heel, you might use it as a brake, drivng your weight into the ground and causing a jarring impact to race upward through your entire leg. In that case, landing mid-foot would be vastly preferred, placing your center of gravity directly through the center of your body, evenly distributing any jarring impact, and allowing you to immediately push forward from your back quadricep.

The bottom line is that running in optimal fashion requires you to pay attention to your natural body mechanics, and to make adjustments when it makes ergonomic sense.

Running uphill and downhill demands some adjustments. Hill running, easily duplicated on a treadmill, is particularly valuable for strengthening the lower leg muscles, gluteals and quadriceps. Uphill training also will also reduce the pounding your knees and other joints endure. Running downhill is another matter entirely. You should concentrate on striding a little longer, in order to maintain better control as gravity pushes you downward. On the other hand, if you stride too far you will be forced to work harder to slow down and regain control. Along with striding a bit longer, you will find it easier to run downhill if you are leaning slightly forward.

If you are competitively racing, you will want to take advantage of that downhill and lean forward a bit more. Of course, this causes your body to undergo a tremendous amount of pounding, but that's the price racers sometimes pay.

When running, respond to your body's needs and demands. That means drinking plenty of fluids, preferably water. If you wait to drink until you are thirsty, then it's probably too late to catch up on your body's immediate needs. So keep hydrated. A good rule of thumb is to drink 8 ounces of water before your run and then to take sips of water at intervals during your workout.

The same goes for other nutritional requirements. Too many people who have taken up running in order to lose weight, starve themselves in conjunction with exercising. Your body needs to be strong and healthy in order to gain the most from your training, and that means being well nourished. Eat a well-balanced diet, a subject that we address in greater detail in Chapter 9.

These are just guidelines. It isn't easy to check or change your form from reading a book. You need to have a coach or friend take a look, or run alongside a building with reflecting windows, so you can see for yourself. In addition, look out for other signs that your form isn't everything it might be, such as tight hamstrings, a sore neck or tender shoulders.

Internal "Form"

Although we have talked about placing your arms here and your feet there, don't become too obsessed with achieving perfection. Addressing form is addressing physical issues. It is also necessary to address your running psychology, your "internal form."

While many people approach workouts with anticipation and even glee, many others do so with, at best, grudging resignation, or, at worst, dread and fear. Attitude counts in every facet of life, especially in exercise. Try optimism. Try a little gleeful anticipation. It shouldn't be that hard — after all, you're doing yourself a good turn, you're doing something that will help you better enjoy many aspects of your life.

And if that doesn't add up to fun, then what does?

Running, at its essence, is natural, the motion free, flowing and easy. This wonderful freedom is what makes running fun.

Optimism, good cheer, hope — key tickets to success in any endeavor. We can't stress enough the importance of adopting a positive mental attitude. This doesn't mean abandoning reason. Be realistic as you approach your treadmill sessions. It is great to imagine yourself running a marathon; just make sure you're methodically preparing and planning to actually achieve the goal. Always consult a doctor before beginning any exercise program, and make sure your goals are appropriate given your physical condition. See to it that your equipment is up to par. As a runner, that's fairly easy—you need a good pair of shoes, and of course a proper treadmill.

When you're exercising, keep track of your pulse before, during and after your run. This doesn't mean you have to keep two fingers plastered to your carotid artery, it just means you should take inventory now and then to ensure that you are working out hard enough without overdoing it. In no time, you'll learn the range of your pulse rate, from resting to exhaustion, and you'll have a better command of how hard you should exercise, and when you should rest.

Rest is an important part of every exercise program. You need to know when to relax and take it easy, for the sake of both your body and your mind. Your body requires time to heal microscopic tears and wounds, to soothe aching joints, to build more muscle. Competitive athletes have long understood the necessity of what is called "stressing and resting." Stressing refers to working hard, which causes cellular changes in the skeletal muscle cells, including nutrient depletion and lactic acid build-up, and torn and swollen cell walls. After a little time off with reduced activity, the lactic acid will be removed, the cells restocked with nutrients and the walls rebuilt stronger than ever. That's how you build more resilient, more powerful muscles — stress and rest. One without the other doesn't work.

Your mind requires time off as well, away from the unending routine, and from thinking about your goals and your pains. You need a break from not only the physical demands but also the mental demands of working out. Whether it's work or working out we've all had the experience of taking a respite and coming back refreshed, ready, and revitalized.

Strategies To Stay Motivated

You can try various strategies to both relax and stimulate yourself during the course of training—"to keep it interesting." One great strategy is to take full advantage of the programs on the console of your treadmill. Today, most treadmills have courses of differing duration and difficulty programmed into the machines, allowing you to choose not only

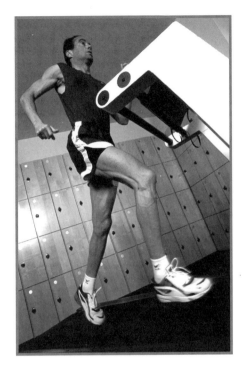 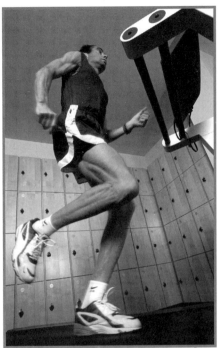

how many minutes you will run, but also how far, at what grade, and how fast. Some courses are designed specifically for walking, and typically feature shifting to higher elevations in order to get the desired training effect. The higher your elevation, whether walking or running, the more hip deflection (the angle of rotation of the hip joint) you incur, and the more gluteal recruitment will be incorporated. You work your butt and thighs more intensely when working on high elevations than when walking or running on a flat surface.

Running programs also frequently give the user the option of interval training, which means alternating periods of high exertion with ones of lower intensity. Interval training can be both quite tiring and extremely effective, helping you to reach greater heights of cardiovascular fitness.

In general, treadmill courses are geared to weight reduction or cardio training. They can tell you how much oxygen you are expending or how many calories you are burning or how many steps you are taking. They can record your favorite courses and track your progress over time.

The configuration of courses and training options that you can find on a treadmill console is virtually inexhaustible. If you happen to be among those people who find exercise repetitive and boring, these options can help keep you interested and entertained. And even if you're not in that group, courses can spare you the trouble of figuring out an effective training routine each time you step on the treadmill, by offering you a variety of instantaneous choices such as hills and valleys, speed work and less strenuous interludes. Programs can distract you, excite you and present you with a new challenge each time you work out. For many people, programs work. Give them a try.

Another motivational strategy is to maintain a log of your exercise sessions that is both reactive and anticipatory. It is reactive when you note how long or how far you ran, your speed, how you felt, and other aspects of a completed run that you might view as important. This record of your training can be useful in several ways: it provides a history of your runs, which will help you understand how you have reached your current level of training and fitness; if you are ever injured, it may reveal where you have over-stressed your body, so you can avoid similar problems in the future; it also can help you plan for your future goals, by giving you a grasp on how you should increase or decrease your training in order to achieve them.

The anticipatory component of the log is equally important, for it allows you to take the time to stop and think about what you want to accomplish, where you want to be going with your exercise. After writing down your goals, you can measure your progress and revise them as you learn through experience what works and what doesn't. This part of the log will help you stay somewhat on track if outside factors, such as injury or increased family or work responsibilities, distract you from your training.

The Five Stages Of Running

Jeff Galloway, a member of the 1972 U.S. Olympic team and perhaps the leading running coach in the country, has identified five stages of running: the beginner, the jogger, the competitor, the athlete, and the runner. He has done so in order to explain the progression that many people experience in the course of their running careers, whatever their individual aspirations. In this way, he reveals the opportunities and obstacles that virtually every runner faces.

The beginner encounters both the exhilaration of starting something new and the fear and pain of what that new experience will bring. He (or she) has decided to change his life by changing his lifestyle, by adopting new habits and commitments, and perhaps shedding a few as well. The demands on the beginner, in time, in effort, in sweat, can quickly become considerable, especially when the reality of the exertion overpowers the thrill of the new.

So many things seem to conspire to get in the way of embarking on a running program. Family and friends might object to the time the beginner is devoting to his new activity. Changes in the weather or work or a thousand other factors can inhibit or interfere with training. Aches and pains scream to slow down, give up, STOP!

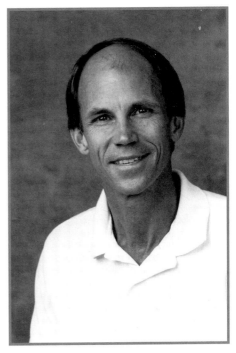

Jeff Galloway

However, if the beginner can make his way past these challenges, if he can overcome the emotional uncertainties and physical strain of his new endeavor, he might, after just a few weeks, find a new comfortable pace and a sense of security in his running routine. And then he will go on, continuing to train.

One of the secrets at this stage is for the beginner to refrain from putting too much pressure on himself. He must not expect too much in the way of fast results. Running is not a quick fix for getting into shape, lowering your cholesterol, or losing weight. Running will accomplish all of these things and more, but it takes time. The beginner has to be conscientious and patient.

In getting started, the beginner often undergoes the same cycle that afflicts those not trying to start but rather to stop a practice, such as smoking, and overeating. They try and fail, and try and fail again. The ones that eventually succeed are those that keep trying until the program sticks.

If and when the beginner sticks to running long enough, he will be ready in short order to move on to the next level.

The jogger has made it past the beginning stage and feels increasingly comfortable with his new discipline. He might enter some local races—5 and 10Ks—though he usually doesn't have a long-range plan or goal. He enjoys running with his friends, though he is sufficiently committed to running whether he is alone or with a group.

If the jogger has to miss a training session, he feels bad or guilty, and imagines that he has taken a step backward. If an injury occurs that sidelines him for some time, the jogger could quit running, or decide to come back stronger. In other words, though he is dedicated, he is not yet as dedicated as he might imagine.

As the jogger's commitment to running deepens, he might very well discover that his competitive spirit, perhaps long buried, has begun to re-emerge. If that should happen, the jogger can be transformed into the competitor.

Competition can be a healthy thing. It can stimulate interest in an activity, it can thrill and excite, it can provide welcome and fun goals.

On the other hand, competition can be a distraction, a negative incentive. It can disappoint and derail from more important objectives.

The jogger who becomes the competitor — and not everyone does, for many people are content to remain at the jogging stage — finds that he is pushing his running harder and harder in order to increase speed and stamina so that he will perform better when racing. He might be reading more running magazines and books, looking for new training techniques, new diets, new shoes — new anything to provide an edge. He will run more races, and measure the progress in his times and distances.

It is not uncommon that his expectations will exceed his progress, and he will become frustrated, demanding more from his training, pushing to his limit and beyond, and cutting short recovery time. Injury is a common possibility at this point, and the competitor will disdain the recommended recovery time in order to begin training again, which threatens to render the injury that much more serious.

The competitor might find that his somewhat obsessive behavior is impinging on other aspects of his life. He talks about running a little bit too much for his non-running (and maybe even his running) family and friends. When a race or training session doesn't go well, he can be rather annoying to be around.

Nonetheless, assuming he survives all the ups and downs of his new running career, and continues to run despite setbacks and injuries and whatnot, the competitor might eventually come to terms with his abilities and goals and move on to the next level: the athlete.

The athlete is more reasonably directed than the competitor. He plans long-term, perhaps six to nine months out, and doesn't run in every race in town, but picks and chooses the ones he finds most appealing. He seeks to do well in each race, same as the competitor, but is more interested in the quality of his performance rather than on a simple measure of time or finishing position. The athlete is more internally directed, and can be completely satisfied by completing a race even below his projected time if he feels he has done his best and enjoyed the effort. The athlete is not in a rush; he may set ambitious goals regarding his running, but he is content to reach them in whatever time frame it may require.

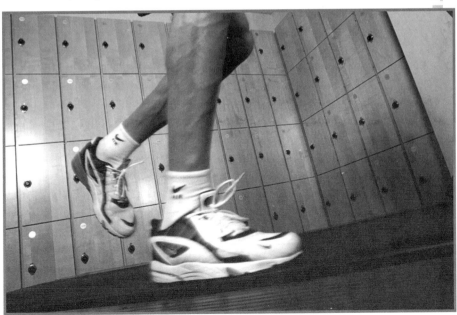

In short, rather than judging success by an absolutely tangible measure, the athlete places it within the context of his larger expectations and experience. As such, he can extract a bit of success from every race or training session.

Many athletes choose to stop competing at all, or take a step back and reduce their training to a readily attainable level. Others find themselves jumping back into the competitive stage for a time, before regaining some equilibrium. The paths are many. One of these paths leads to the last stage, that of the runner.

The runner has reached a place where all the elements of running are balanced in his life. Running has become as natural and integrated a part of his existence as eating or sleeping. It is what he does for a certain time during the day. In this manner, running is not the most important thing in his life, it does not crowd out family or friends or work. Running is simply part of who the runner is, and as such, he runs.

Sometimes he set goals, and competes in a race. Other times — more often, in fact—he runs alone, enjoying the solitude, the chance to feel his body in motion, relishing the inner peace the activity inspires.

If injury occurs, the runner has no problem resting until it is completely healed, allowing him to return to the track or treadmill in fine shape, so he truly can appreciate each session. He has combined the best of all the stages of running: the excitement of the beginner, the enthusiasm of the jogger, the purposefulness of the competitor, the internal exploration of the athlete. In doing so, he has emerged as a complete runner and more interesting, more involved, content human being.

One or all of Jeff Galloway's five stages may correspond to your view or yourself, or your definition of running. Take a moment to see if you can locate yourself on the scale, and then determine where you really want to be. You may find this a useful exercise.

We are going to hear more from Jeff in the chapter after next, as we rely upon him to talk about marathon training. We focus on the marathon in Chapter 8 because this ultimate race, which is both so difficult and so doable, brings into play so many aspects of training. Talking about the marathon demands that we be as specific as possible, because every step counts when you're thinking about running 26 miles.

And if you're not completely convinced of the logic behind this concentration on the marathon, don't despair — the next chapter features several shorter running programs from Alberto Salazar, which you should find intriguing and useful.

Whether you never intend to run a marathon, or plan to complete one a week in the next year, the following two chapters contain some tips and ideas that you should find useful.

Some of this information is based on Jeff's book *Marathon!* ©2000. Published by Phidippides Publications. For more information visit Jeff's website at **www.jeffgalloway.com**.

CHAPTER 7

Running: Alberto's Way

ALBERTO SALAZAR IS A PRACTICAL FELLOW. As a professional runner, he has to be — he has to know how to push his body without injuring it, he has to hold no illusions about how fast and how far he must run to gain his desired results. There are few delusions possible because the measure for a professional runner is easily quantified in distance covered and times achieved. Unlike in other activities, the runner is not an individual within a team framework, where allowances must be made for the mistakes or abilities of others. Rather, the runner is an individual who in reality is competing against himself.

In this chapter, Alberto provides training programs both for beginners and advanced runners.

Beginner's Program

One key to remember: If you're looking for a 30-minute program, incorporate the warm-up and cool-down into the routine. Otherwise, you won't have sufficient time to exercise. (If you warmed up and cooled down for a mile, that would only leave about 15 minutes for the actual workout!) Instead, start your exercise session slowly, work up to the desired intensity level, then back down to an easier pace at the end of your workout.

The following workout can be completed in 30 minutes, or extended for a couple of hours. You just have to figure out

1 how far you want to run in total; and

2 your starting pace, which must be slow enough to be quite comfortable, and allows you to both slow down and speed up without undue strain.

The Workout:

PHASE 1

- Start at a brisk walking pace—4.0 MPH is recommended (approx.15:00 per mile.)
- Speed up to 14:00 per mile pace for a quarter-mile. This is a little more than a walk.
- Slow back down to walking a quarter-mile at a 15:00 pace.
- Speed back up to 14:00 mile pace for a quarter-mile. Continue this for 30 to 40 minutes, which should add up to about 2.25 to 2.75 miles.
- Do this 4 to 6 times per week for three weeks.

PHASE 2

- Keeping the walking pace the same for every other quarter-mile, alternate it with jogging a quarter at a 13:00 mile pace. It's not very different from Phase 1, just a little faster, moving from a fast walk to a slow jog.
- Do this 4 to 6 times per week for three weeks.

PHASE 3

- Increase the jogging pace to a 12:00 pace, while keeping the walking pace at 15:00 per mile. Exercise for 30 to 40 minutes.
- Do this 4 to 6 times per week for three weeks.
- After that, keep dropping the quarter-mile jogging pace by 1:00 per mile until you get to a 10:00 per mile pace. Maintain that pace for three weeks, doing the workout 4 to 6 times per week.

PHASE 4

Okay. You're training at a quite decent pace, and now you're ready for an alteration in the routine. Your next round of improvement will not come by accelerating your running pace—you're going at an efficient clip—but rather, by changing the distance you run.

- Thus, the next training session will have you starting off by walking a quarter-mile at a 15:00 pace. Then you'll jog four-tenths of a mile (.4 mile) at a slightly slower pace than the previous three-week cycle—let's say an 11:00 mile pace.
- Walk a quarter-mile at a 15:00 pace.
- Jog the next .4 mile at the 11:00 pace. Continue alternating between walking and jogging for 30 to 40 minutes.
- Do this schedule 4 to 6 times per week for three weeks.

PHASE 5

- During your next phase, increase the jogging pace to 10:30 per mile for each .4 mile segment. Keep the walking portions the same in distance and speed.
- Do this 4 to 6 times per week for three weeks.
- Increase the jogging pace to 10:00 per mile for each .4 mile. Do this 4 to 6 times per week for three weeks.

PHASE 6

- Now it's time for another shift. Increase the jogging distance to a half-mile, while keeping the walking part the same. If you have to, slow down your pace to 10:30 and work up to 10:00. If you feel good, start off at 10:00. Either way, once you've done three weeks of jogging .5 mile at a 10:00 pace, you're ready to change the walking portion.

PHASE 7

- Alternate walking only .15 mile at a 15:00 pace, with jogging .5 miles at a 10:00 pace for 30 to 40 minutes. Again, do this 4 to 6 times per week for three weeks.

PHASE 8

- Drop the walking segment down to a mere tenth of a mile (.1 mile), undertaken at the familiar 15:00 pace. This means that you're only going to walk for about a minute and half. Alternate with jogging a half-mile at a 10:00 pace—or even faster if it feels comfortable. Do this 4 to 6 times per week for three weeks.

PHASE 9

- Drop the walking distance down to .5 mile, at the 15:00 pace. That adds up to only 45 seconds of walking. Jog at the 10:00 pace for a half-mile, before returning to the walking segment, and then back to jogging. Do this 4 to 6 times per week for three weeks.

PHASE 10—YOU'RE THERE!

Okay. We're ready for the final segment, which is simplicity itself. Drop the walking altogether and run continuously at the 10:00 pace for 30 to 40 minutes.

Now you're running, without pausing, stopping or interruption. This training course requires approximately six months to complete. That might seem like a long time to reach this point, but it's a smart, safe way to avoid injury, and frustration and to accomplish your goals.

You can go on like this, or return to interspersing some slow jogging instead of walking, into your program, particularly if you want to use this system to improve your speed. Begin by alternating jogging quarter-mile segments at a 10:00 pace, with quarter-mile segments at a 9:30 pace. Back and forth you go, until you've done your 30 to 40 minutes. Once you've done this for three weeks, quicken your pace, working your way to an 8:30 pace.

Once you've conquered that, start increasing the distance during the 8:30 pace, while decreasing the distance of the slow jogging portion, in the manner described previously, until you can run for 30 to 40 minutes at the 8:30 pace.

Advanced Training Sessions

As a world-class runner, Alberto knows how to improve his performance. In the following more advanced Training Sessions, he shares some good interval training ideas with those of you who are ready for a new challenge.

Training Session 1

We begin with one of Alberto's personal favorite workouts, which we'll call Training Session 1. Because it is his very own routine, Alberto will explain it to you directly.

"One of the treadmill's greatest attributes is the runner's absolute command of its functions. This allows you to do your warm-up gradually and consistently, accelerating as you see fit. What I like to do is simply incorporate the warm-up into the workout. This both saves time and grants me the ability to warm-up perfectly in order to reach that session's ultimate speed goal.

One of my favorite workouts is a continuous 6-8 mile run. I start out at what I call my base pace or recovery pace, which is currently a 7:03 per mile pace. I run some 220 yards at that pace, which works out to .12–.13 miles on the treadmill. Then, I pick up the pace by .1 MPH. On my Precor machine, I accomplish this by pressing the speed button once, which increases the speed to about 6:58 per mile pace.

I run at that speed for .12–.13 miles, which brings my total to a full quarter-mile. I slow down to my recovery pace by pressing the appropriate button once.

I run another .12 mile at the recovery pace. Next, I increase the speed by running the next .12 miles at a 6:53 mile pace, (accomplished by pressing the speed button twice).

After that, I slow back down to my 7:03 pace. I do another .12 mile, then speed up to 6:49.

The idea is that I'm very gradually running faster and faster for every other .12 mile run, but then return to my steady recovery pace.

After sticking to this course for approximately 3–4 miles, I then start back up in reverse order. That means that while my fastest .12 mile on the way down was a 5:00 mile pace, as I start on my way back up this training regimen, I lead off with a 5:02. Between each of these faster .12 miles, I continue to run my recovery 7:03 pace.

By the time I'm finished, I've done what I'd call a nice Fartlek workout. [Fartlek is similar to interval training, consisting of work-rest intervals that usually are determined by how a participant feels. The term Fartlek is Swedish for speed play, which of course assumes anybody would consider running a 5-minute mile pace playing.]

To figure out your own recovery pace, which is the pace with which you would start out, calculate the pace at which you run or might conceive of running a marathon (If a marathon is inconceivable, use your time for a 10K race) and then add 30 seconds per mile. For example if you can run a 7 minute (7:00) mile, your recovery pace should be 7:30.

I'm working my way back into shape now. I'm running anywhere from 6:00 to 6:30 for my recovery pace, and cutting down to about a 4:40 pace, with my average pace coming close to 6:00.

Why, just the other day, I did a 20 miler at a 6:45 recovery pace and cut down to 4:40, and ended up running an average of 5:57 for the whole distance.

You can see that although the recovery pace may seem very easy at first, the further you go with this workout, the more you'll need to recover as you run faster and faster.

The best part is that the training tends to go very quickly mentally because you're always changing the pace, always keeping it interesting, always keeping it fun. What also will keep it interesting and fun for you is that this is a completely flexible program that can be applied to any length run, short or long."

Training Session 2

"Here's another type of Fartlek-type workout. I start out at an easy pace—say, 7:30 in my case—and every .12 mile I pick it up by pushing the speed button once, which effectively quickens the pace by about 3 to 4 seconds. The difference between this and the prior workout is that you never, ever slow down, you're always speeding up.

I keep picking up the pace to until I start to feel uncomfortable, until I'm pretty sure I can't speed up much more. At that point, I start head-ing in the other direction, slowing down the pace every .12 mile. You don't get a recovery in this workout, so the workout will be more intense albeit shorter. Consequently, this schedule might be better suited for a 5K or 10K, rather than a marathon.

I like this one a lot. It can be tough, but well worth the effort."

Training Session 3

Training Session 3 is more of a standard interval schedule, where you run repeat half-miles. Start with your current marathon pace—let's peg it at an 8:00 mile pace—and divide that in half to conform to our half-mile schedule. That's 4:00. Run your first half-mile at 4:00, then jog at about a 10:00 pace for a quarter-mile.

Run the next half-mile in 3:55, which is equal to a 7:50 mile pace.

Back up to a 10:00 pace for a quarter-mile.

Shave another 10 seconds off the pace, which means you run the next half-mile in 3:50.

Keep progressing in this manner, until you can't run at a faster pace.

At the point, you have two options.

The first is better suited to preparing for a 10K. Alter your distance so that you're running a quarter-mile for your next interval, instead of a half-mile. You will still take that quarter-mile to recover.

In this scenario, each quarter-mile will be run at .1 mile per hour faster, so if you're last half was run at 6:40, for instance, your next quarter will be a 6:36 pace, followed by 6:33, so on. When you can't run any faster for a quarter, start running .12–.13 miles, 220 yards, while still taking the quarter-mile recovery run.

You see how cruel—uh, efficient—this is? Just when you think you're done, we pull you back in. We work you harder, squeezing the very last bit of energy from your bones and muscles.

When you can't run those 220s any faster, then you get down on your hands and knees and crawl. Just kidding. The .12s are the last stop on this session.

The second option is designed for marathon preparation. When you've gone as far as you can go with the half-milers, start doing each successive half-mile a little slower. How much slower is up to you — as long as you stay within a 5 to 10 second range.

By slowing down in this progressive fashion, you can run farther, and, yes, wring every ounce of strength from you.

• • •

Alberto has this to say about this trio of workouts: "What I really like about these workouts is that you pick up the pace very gradually, which distracts the runner from fretting about the workout and perhaps chickening out. You don't really start hurting for a while, and by then, mentally, you're often psyched up about how much you've already done. You feel you've been through the worst of it, and you've got to hold on for only a bit more."

That attitude about exercise and training, is one big factor, (apart from talent), that separates world-class athletes from the rest of humanity.

• • •

All of the sessions in this chapter are custom-made for the treadmill, because they require precision of pace and distance. And make no mistake: Nothing in this chapter can be billed as anything other than hardcore and demanding, requiring dedication and patience. But that's how Alberto sees it, and that's how he lives it.

Many of you appreciate this outlook. Many will absolutely enjoy lacing up those sneakers and following our champ's recommendations, sweat and strain be damned.

Some of you are already looking for another type of running program or a plan work to up to running long distance races such as marathons.

If you're one of those people, your prayers are about to be answered.

CHAPTER 8

Running: The Nitty-Gritty of Training for a Marathon From Beginner to Advanced

IN CHAPTER 6 WE INTRODUCED YOU to Jeff Galloway's Five Stages of Running. It is important to know more about Jeff before reading this chapter, so you will understand why he can help you achieve your goals, whatever they may be. Jeff is a navy veteran with a master's degree in social studies. He was a member of the 1972 U.S. Olympic team, qualifying for the 10,000-meter event. He set an American record for 10 miles one year later, and ran for the United States as a member of the national team in Europe, Russia and Africa.

He founded Phidippides, now a nationally franchised chain of running stores, runs fitness vacation camps in California, Colorado and British Columbia, and gives lectures and clinics on running throughout the world.

It's obvious that as an athlete, educator and entrepreneur, Jeff knows what he's talking about when it comes to running and fitness.

But there's more. In the mid-Seventies, as he entered his thirties, Jeff began to devise a new exercise routine that called for less weekly mileage than was the norm for distance race training, and was punctuated by a long run every other week. Over time, he refined this new way of training and at the age 35, he ran his fastest marathon ever, completing the Houston-Tenneco Marathon in 2:16:35.

That extraordinary marathon result is the key to this chapter. For Jeff uncovered a system for training that can benefit everyone who steps on a treadmill, whether or not you want to run a marathon. Of course, more than 100,000 people have used Jeff's methods to run and compete in a marathon, so if you're interested in going all the way, here's your chance to learn from the best.

Before we delve into Jeff's ideas and plans, remember to be smart and safe. As we've said before, whenever you start any exercise program, you must make sure you're medically capable of going beyond your current level of exertion. When you do embark upon a program, build your training gradually, ensuring that you don't push too far or injure yourself. If you do sustain an injury of any sort, give yourself time to heal, and see a doctor or therapist if necessary to speed your recovery.

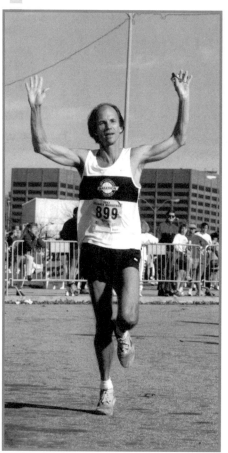

Jeff Galloway

Remember that any advice you glean from a book or clinic is targeted to a broad audience and you might have to modify it to suit your individual needs. Also keep in mind that achieving results through exercise takes time and patience.

And finally—though more appropriately first and foremost—don't forget to have fun!

Now, having gotten the preliminaries out of the way, let's begin.

We were meant to run. It is part of our evolutionary birthright, an important component to how we tracked and hunted, how we migrated and triumphed, how we populated a planet and emerged as the most successful species on earth.

We have kept moving forward for 100,000 years of human survival. Moving forward swiftly is so essential a part of our make-up that we instinctively feel a measure of security when we move in response to stress or danger, whether that response means pacing or fleeing, marching or fighting. Some sorts of insects and animals respond to trouble by freezing and staying absolutely still. Human beings respond by acting.

In stark contrast, and for the first time in human history, the technology of civilization has rendered most of us sedentary. Many of us have forgone our natural abilities and urges because of cars, televisions, remote controls, elevators and the myriad other conveniences (sometimes annoyances) of modern life.

So we miss exercise. We miss running, whether we are aware of it or not, whether we want to believe it or not. And when we do run and fill our lungs and work our muscles, we begin to feel right, somehow in tune with the world and ourselves. We intuitively understand this is the way it was meant to be. That is, of course, assuming we're not overwhelmed by oxygen deficiency, as we gasp for air, or are consumed by the pain radiating from our neglected limbs. Once we get past that, many of us are surprised to discover a new joy and freedom and strength emanating from within. Therefore, it is imperative that we exercise enough to get beyond that initial pain, or, even better, that we exercise in a manner that ensures that we won't unnecessarily stress or damage our body, but rather build our strength slowly, carefully and intelligently.

> **A general rule: If you've never exercised, and you're going out there without a specific program, think about walking five minutes for every minute of jogging.**

The payoff to training smart can be instantaneous. Even an accomplished athlete like Jeff Galloway has benefited from altering his training patterns. Only a few years ago, after years of running hard and fast, training in the tough mode practiced by virtually all top athletes, he re-evaluated his program, and shifted from an every-other-day schedule to running two days out of three. In addition, he slowed down all of his runs. The reason he changed was simple—to avoid stress and injury, which had afflicted him throughout his career,—and the benefits were several. As Jeff writes in his groundbreaking book, **Marathon!**:

Prior to this slowdown, I had been starting my runs on slow days at 7-7:30 minutes per mile. When I shifted into "slow" gear, the pace became about 9-10 minutes per mile. Yes, even though I still run some 10K races at 5:30 pace, I start virtually all of my daily runs at about 10 minutes per mile and feel great because of it.

The unexpected benefit of this extra slow start has been an early shift into the right brain. Much sooner than usual, I found my mind wandering into creative journeys of all types. When the body is not under the usual stress of starting exercise at "normal" pace, it will relax, and your left brain doesn't have to respond to stress with its usual stream of negative messages.

Most folks go too fast in the beginning of a run because their pacing instincts take over. It's easy to go too fast before the body is warmed up because the biomechanics of running form allow us to move along very efficiently at a pace that is too fast for the muscles, the energy resources, and the cardiovascular system. A gentle warm-up will gradually introduce the muscles and all of your system to exercise at the same time.

When in doubt, run slower at the beginning. You'll increase your enjoyment without significantly lowering the training effect or the fat-burning.

Jeff offers up a few concepts that call for reviewing.

First off, even with Jeff's slowdown, he's still moving faster than most of us. Nonetheless, the basics underlying what works for him can work for all of us.

He talks about the right brain versus the left brain. It has long been established that the left side of the brain is your center of logic and reason, while the right side determines creativity and intuition. When something goes wrong, or you are under stress, the left brain responds in a negative fashion, coming up with excuses and problems, etc. When stress is reduced, the right brain takes over, and can derive original, perceptive, clear-sighted solutions to almost anything.

Jeff is really talking not about running, but about you, and what motivates—and inhibits—your running, as well as everything else in your life. When specifically applied to running, we must grasp that running is as much in your mind as your legs, and your mind's response to stimuli and stress can help or hurt your training.

Delving more into the physical aspect of running, Jeff discovered that starting slower and maintaining a slower than usual pace has allowed his body to properly warm-up while not reducing the fat-burning benefits that so many of us want to attain.

By going slower, which both protects his legs and engages his right brain, Jeff is clearly enjoying his running considerably more than before, physically, intellectually and emotionally.

The Programs

The beginners among you, the as-of-today non-runners, might be feeling a mixture of impatience and anxiety at this point. Enough of the health benefits of running! Enough about the sheer joy of spreading your wings and soaring, albeit without leaving the ground! Enough good cheer!

Let's get running.

No problem. Jeff Galloway designed the accompanying training schedule for beginners, who may or may not have any interest in working up to marathon distance. Immediately following the schedule is a discussion of many of its main points.

Enjoy.

The Beginner Program

Though the schedule is 29 weeks long, you don't have to follow through to the end, especially if you have reached a running level and distance that you feel is just right for you, your goals, your interest, your abilities.

Let's talk pace, and for you beginners, that means maintaining a running speed that enables you to talk throughout your training session. Being conversational does not mean you have to have a debate while exercising; rather, it means not having to suck down huge draughts of oxygen in between every word.

In examining the schedule, you will note that you will be doing more walking than running, especially in the earlier weeks. Walking is a key component of every Galloway schedule, and the reasons are self-evident—at least once Jeff explains them.

To quote Jeff: "The human body wasn't designed for running continuously for long distances." This is not to say that people don't do it. Consider the original marathoner, the noble Athenian, Phidippides. In 490 B.C., the Athenians defeated the invading Persians on the Plain of Marathon. Since the militaristic, marauding Persians outnumbered the small, volunteer army of the democratic city-state five to one, this victory was rather unexpected. In order to stop their fellow Athenians from burning and abandoning the city, the Athenian generals dispatched Phidippides to run home and tell the citizens the good news. Phidippides was the logical choice. After all, not long before he had raced to Sparta—130 miles in a day and half—to request some assistance from the extremely tough Spartans.

After not only fighting the whole day against the Persians, but also suffering a wound, Phidippides ran the 25 miles or so back to Athens. As history tells us, he told the people of the victory, and then expired. That's right—he died, dropped dead right on the spot.

Not exactly the greatest recommendation for an event that's supposed to be fun for the whole family.

Running these far distances isn't necessarily the best thing for your body. Don't get us wrong—running is definitely good—but running mile after mile can wreak havoc your knees, hips and feet. This is not to say you shouldn't do it—this is to say that you should do it right.

And right means including some walking, especially if you're just starting out on your exercise program. If you aren't accustomed to running, repetitively using the main running muscles in exactly the same way, will quickly cause them to fatigue and may lead to damage. However, if you shift some of the work being done by the forward motion muscles by walking, you'll continue to improve your conditioning while reducing the strain on your muscles. In addition, the shifting will actually increase total muscle capacity by using more of the resources and reserves inside your muscles.

Start easy. A general rule: If you've never exercised, and do not have a specific program, think about walking five minutes for every minute

Beginner's Program

Weeks 1 – 29

	Mon	Tues	Wed	Thurs	Fri	Sat	Sun
1	walk 30	run/walk 30	walk 30	run/walk 30	walk 30	off	3–4 miles run/walk
2	walk 30	run/walk 30	walk 30	run/walk 30	walk 30	off	4–5 miles run/walk
3	walk 30	run/walk 30	walk 30	run/walk 30	walk 30	off	5–6 miles run/walk
4	walk 30	run/walk 30	walk 30	run/walk 30	walk 30	off	6–7 miles run/walk
5	walk 30	run/walk 30	walk 30	run/walk 30	walk 30	off	7–8 miles run/walk
6	walk 30	run/walk 30	walk 30	run/walk 30	walk 30	off	8–9 miles
7	walk 30	run/walk 30	walk 30	run/walk 30	walk 30	off	9–10 miles
8	walk 30	run/walk 30	walk 30	run/walk 30	walk 30	off	10–11 miles
9	walk 30	run/walk 30	walk 30	run/walk 30	walk 30	off	11–12 miles
10	walk 30	run/walk 30	walk 30	run/walk 30	walk 30	off	6 miles
11	walk 30	run/walk 30	walk 30	run/walk 30	walk 30	off	13–14 miles
12	walk 30	run/walk 30	walk 30	run/walk 30	walk 30	off	7 miles
13	walk 30	run/walk 30	walk 30	run/walk 30	walk 30	off	15–16 miles
14	walk 30	run/walk 30	walk 30	run/walk 30	walk 30	off	7 miles
15	walk 30	run/walk 30	walk 30	run/walk 30	walk 30	off	17–18 miles
16	walk 30	run/walk 30	walk 30	run/walk 30	walk 30	off	8 miles
17	walk 30	run/walk 30	walk 30	run/walk 30	walk 30	off	19–20 miles
18	walk 30	run/walk 30	walk 30	run/walk 30	walk 30	off	8–9 miles
19	walk 30	run/walk 30	walk 30	run/walk 30	walk 30	off	8–9 miles
20	walk 30	run/walk 30	walk 30	run/walk 30	walk 30	off	22–23 miles
21	walk 30	run/walk 30	walk 30	run/walk 30	walk 30	off	8–10 miles
22	walk 30	run/walk 30	walk 30	run/walk 30	walk 30	off	8–10 miles
23	walk 30	run/walk 30	walk 30	run/walk 30	walk 30	off	24–26 miles
24	walk 30	run/walk 30	walk 30	run/walk 30	walk 30	off	8–10 miles
25	walk 30	run/walk 30	walk 30	run/walk 30	walk 30	off	8–10 miles
26	walk 30	off	walk 30	off	walk 30	off	**THE MARATHON**
27	walk 45	run/walk 45	walk 30–60	run/walk 40	walk 30–60	off	7–10 miles run/walk
28	walk 45	run/walk 45	walk 30–60	run/walk 45	walk 30–60	off	9–15 miles run/walk
29	walk 45	run/walk 45	walk 30–60	run/walk 45	walk 30–60	off	12–20 miles run/walk

of jogging. As you get in better shape, shave a minute off the walking and tack it onto the jogging. Improve some more and do the same again.

This is not to imply that you eventually give up the walking part of the equation, but you certainly can, especially if your goal is to stick to running anywhere between 2–5 miles, 3–5 days a week.

For those of you who will follow the beginner's schedule laid out above, walking is one of the essential elements. On every "run/walk" day you find on Tuesday and Thursday, and sometimes on Sunday, walk for 2–3 minutes and jog for 1-2 minutes. Every 3–4 weeks, review your progress. If you wish, you can increase your running by altering the equation to running for 2 minutes and then walking for 3 minutes. If that eventually becomes too easy for you, move on towards an equilibrium, by running for two minutes and walking for two minutes.

As you increase your mileage, be sure to drink plenty of water, keep your blood sugar up by taking in enough nutrients via fruits, athletic supplements and nutritional bars before and during training.

This is the beginner's program. Take it as far as you wish. Stop at any time when you've reached a point where you're content with the state of your exercise program.

On the other hand, many of you will want to continue intensifying your training, even preparing for a marathon that's out there somewhere, waiting for you like the great white whale was waiting for Captain Ahab.

For those in that category, let's move along.

Major Components of
Jeff Galloway's Marathon Training Schedule

Incorporate the following techniques into your training sessions and you'll be well on your way to Marathon success:

- Cross Training (varying the mode of your workout)
- 5K Races (short, fast races that help get you used to the pressure of racing)
- Hill Work to strengthen leg muscles.
- Mile Repeats (alternating running segments with a walk between, then repeating)
- Acceleration-Gliders (gliding with little effort in a comfortable rhythm to fine tune your running technique)

ONE IMPORTANT NOTE: As you have noticed, we've talked about running slowly and then even more slowly, and that theme will be sounded again in the near future. This does not mean you must learn to run more deliberately or leisurely than usual. However, not having to push to the max, not having to keep your legs churning as furiously as possible, will prove nothing less than liberating to many runners. Of course, you can always go faster, you can always sprint as far as you can stand it, relishing the burn. The point is, you don't have to run yourself into the ground every time you get on the treadmill to have an invigorating, healthy, utterly satisfying running experience.

Marathon Training Schedules

We're concentrating on the marathon because it demands so much from the runner, spurring him to try different training techniques. Even though the event is so demanding, don't let age stop you from trying. Jeff estimates that more than 30 percent of those who use his program to run a marathon are over 50 years old. It is not a question of age, but of preparation, discipline and desire.

Getting to the nitty-gritty, Jeff charts out exactly what the runner should do in order to achieve a certain time in the marathon. We're going to reprint Jeff's program—revolutionary in its approach, as you will see—and then analyze it so you can understand its intricacies.

In *Marathon!*, Jeff provides schedules for runners seeking to finish in a variety of times, from those first-timers hoping to simply finish, without concern for achieving any particular time, to those experienced, exceptional marathoners aiming to complete the race in 2 hours, 39 minutes.

We reproduce just a few of those schedules in order to give you an idea of what it takes to finish the marathon, from easy to oh-so-fast. Within these parameters, you might find the schedule that promises a race that you envision as your consummate performance.

(If you want to get the total sweep of schedules from Jeff, as well as access his entire, inexhaustible encyclopedia of information on running and training, check out his web site at www.jeffgalloway.com.)

"To Finish" Marathon

The first schedule is simply entitled "To Finish" Program, and that is the objective. Time is not a consideration, but rather that the runner complete the course and not suffer unduly doing it, nor suffer to any unnecessary degree in the days following the marathon.

Same as with the beginner's program, try to stay conversational, so you don't push too hard, too soon.

As always, keep hydrated and nutritionally satiated before and during your training, especially during your long runs.

Last, though there is a certain play within the long runs, it is suggested that during week 23, you try to run the entire 26 miles, rather than 24. Emotionally and physically, you will be much better prepared for the marathon if you have already reached that distance in training.

It's that simple. Well, it's not that simple, not really, because you have to put in the time and the miles. But it is that simple when you consider the daily requirements of the schedule, which are straightforward and achievable.

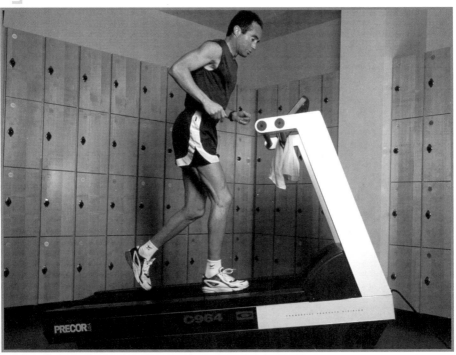

"To Finish" Marathon

Weeks 1 – 29

	Mon	Tues	Wed	Thurs	Fri	Sat	Sun
1	walk/XT 40	run 30–40	walk or XT	run 30–40	walk or XT	off	3 miles easy
2	walk/XT 40	run 30–40	walk or XT	run 30–40	walk or XT	off	4 miles
3	walk/XT 40	run 30–40	walk or XT	run 30–40	walk or XT	off	5 miles
4	walk/XT 40	run 30–40	walk or XT	run 30–40	walk or XT	off	6 miles
5	walk/XT 40	run 30–40	walk or XT	run 30–40	walk or XT	off	7 miles
6	walk/XT 40	run 30–40	walk or XT	run 30–40	walk or XT	off	8 miles
7	walk/XT 40	run 30–40	walk or XT	run 30–40	walk or XT	off	9 miles
8	walk/XT 40	run 30–40	walk or XT	run 30–40	walk or XT	off	10 miles
9	walk/XT 40	run 30–40	walk or XT	run 30–40	walk or XT	off	11–12 miles
10	walk/XT 40	run 30–40	walk or XT	run 30–40	walk or XT	off	6 miles
11	walk/XT 40	run 30–40	walk or XT	run 30–40	walk or XT	off	13–14 miles
12	walk/XT 40	run 30–40	walk or XT	run 30–40	walk or XT	off	7 miles
13	walk/XT 40	run 30–40	walk or XT	run 30–40	walk or XT	off	15–16 miles
14	walk/XT 40	run 30–40	walk or XT	run 30–40	walk or XT	off	8 miles
15	walk/XT 40	run 30–40	walk or XT	run 30–40	walk or XT	off	17–18 miles
16	walk/XT 40	run 30–40	walk or XT	run 30–40	walk or XT	off	8–10 miles
17	walk/XT 40	run 30–40	walk or XT	run 30–40	walk or XT	off	19–20 miles
18	walk/XT 40	run 30–40	walk or XT	run 30–40	walk or XT	off	5k race or 8–10 miles
19	walk/XT 40	run 30–40	walk or XT	run 30–40	walk or XT	off	8–9 miles
20	walk/XT 40	run 30–40	walk or XT	run 30–40	walk or XT	off	22–23 miles
21	walk/XT 40	run 30–40	walk or XT	run 30–40	walk or XT	off	5k race or 8–10 miles
22	walk/XT 40	run 30–40	walk or XT	run 30–40	walk or XT	off	8–10 miles
23	walk/XT 40	run 30–40	walk or XT	run 30–40	walk or XT	off	24–26 miles
24	walk/XT 40	run 30–40	walk or XT	run 30–40	walk or XT	off	5k race or 8–10 miles
25	walk/XT 40	run 30–40	walk or XT	run 30–40	walk or XT	off	8–10 miles
26	run 40	off	run 30	off	run/walk 30	off	**THE MARATHON**
27	Walk 45	run/walk 30	walk 30–60	run/walk 45	run/walk 30–60	off	7–10 miles run/walk
28	Walk 45	run/walk 45	walk 30–60	run/walk 45	run/walk 30–60	off	9–15 miles run/walk
29	Walk 45	run/walk 45	walk 30–60	run/walk 45	run/walk 30–60	off	12–20 miles run/walk

"XT" refers to cross training, and that encompasses doing an activity other than running, such as cycling, swimming, water running, cross-country skiing and elliptical machines (see Chapter 5). The objective is to exercise without enduring the pounding that comes with running.

4:40 Marathon

The following schedule is for those who want to finish the marathon in a time of 4:40. It has more nuances, more variations in speed and in elevation. You will see how your running changes with the change in your goals.

Let's begin by returning to the matter of walking. Walking in the midst of your training runs, particularly the long runs, will improve your training, racing and recovery to an amazing extent. We've already gone through some of the reasons that walking is beneficial. Here's one more: if you do run a marathon, and have run one before, you might find that you improve your time by 10, 20, 30 or more minutes if you include walking breaks.

The breaks, if started early enough and continued for the whole race, will give the primary leg muscles the respite they need to recover sufficiently to keep them resilient and strong to the end of the race.

During training, walking will help extend your training sessions without additional pain, and prepare you for the marathon. Consider the numbers when doing a 20-mile training run, and look how rapidly the formula changes:

If you walk 1 minute every 5 minutes from the beginning, you'll incur only 12 to 13 miles of pounding.

If you walk 1 minute every 10 minutes from the beginning, you'll incur only 14 to 15 miles of pounding.

If you walk 1 minute every 5 minutes starting at mile 5 to 7, you'll incur only 15 to 17 miles of pounding.

If you walk 1 minute every 10 minutes starting at mile 5 to 7, you'll incur only 17 to 19 miles of pounding.

Remember when we said this was simple? Well, those numbers speak volumes in simple terms.

The bottom line is, you do the long runs to build endurance, and breaking up the run with some walking won't reduce the efficacy of your training.

Of all of Jeff's tips, perhaps none will improve your training and racing in every way more than taking walking breaks.

We're going to use only one example from Jeff's catalogue of examples to demonstrate the effectiveness of this strategy. It seems that a

4:40 Marathon

Weeks 1–29

	Mon	Tues	Wed	Thurs	Fri	Sat	Sun
1	XT	40–50	20–30	XT	40–50	off	4–6 hills (5–7 miles)
2	XT	40–50	20–30	XT	40–50	off	5k race (6–7 miles)
3	XT	40–50	20–30	XT	40–50	off	7–8 hills (7–8 miles)
4	XT	40–50	20–30	XT	40–50	off	9–10 hills (8–9 miles)
5	XT	45–50	25–35	XT	45–50	off	5k race (9–10 miles)
6	XT	45–50	25–35	XT	45–50	off	3–4 x 1 mile (11 miles)
7	XT	45–50	25–35	XT	45–50	off	4–5 x 1 mile (8 miles)
8	XT	45–50	25–35	XT	45–50	off	5–6 x 1 mile (13 miles)
9	XT	45–55	25–35	XT	45–50	off	5k race (6 miles)
10	XT	45–55	25–40	XT	45–55	off	15–16 miles easy
11	XT	45–55	25–40	XT	45–55	off	5k race (6 miles)
12	XT	45–55	25–40	XT	45–55	off	17–18 miles easy
13	XT	45–55	25–40	XT	45–55	off	5–6 x 1 mile
14	XT	45–55	25–40	XT	45–55	off	19–20 miles easy
15	XT	45–55	25–40	XT	45–55	off	5k race (10 miles)
16	XT	45–55	25–40	XT	45–55	off	5 x 1 mile
17	XT	45–55	25–40	XT	45–55	off	22–23 miles easy
18	XT	45–55	25–40	XT	45–55	off	5k race
19	XT	45–55	25–40	XT	45–55	off	4 x 1 mile
20	XT	45–55	25–40	XT	45–55	off	24–26 miles easy
21	XT	45–55	25–40	XT	45–55	off	5k race
22	XT	45–55	25–40	XT	45–55	off	3–4 x 1 mile
23	XT	45–55	25–40	XT	45–55	off	27–28 miles easy
24	XT	45–55	25–40	XT	45–55	off	5k or 3 x 1 mile
25	XT	40–45	20–25	XT	40–45	off	3 x 1 mile
26	XT	off	run 30	XT	run 30	off	**THE MARATHON**
27	XT	run/walk 30	walk 30–60	XT	walk 30–60	off	7–10 miles walk–run
28	XT	run/walk 45	walk 30–60	XT	walk 30–60	off	9–15 miles run/walk
29	XT	run/walk 45	walk 30–60	XT	walk 30–60	off	12–20 miles run/walk

friend of Jeff's, a fellow in his late forties, had been endeavoring for years to run a 3:30 marathon. Unfortunately, despite his best efforts, 3:40 was the fastest he could go.

Jeff stepped in to help get his pal over (or under) the hump, and taught him about the walking breaks. He did as he was supposed to in the course of his marathon preparation -- under the tutelage of one of Jeff's trainers—running, walking, running, so on, but he wasn't happy about it. No way. He belittled the walking, as though it wasn't a thing that real runners did.

Come marathon morning, the man's trainer stood beside him and physically forced him to walk for one minute each mile. At mile 18, the trainer released his charge from his bondage with the words, "Well, you seem to have just enough life in your legs so run along now!"

Jeff (Galloway) discovered that starting slower and maintaining a slower than usual pace has allowed his body to properly warm-up while not reducing the fat-burning benefits that so many of us want to attain.

And away the man went, finishing—lo and behold—in 3:25, no less than 15 minutes faster than his fastest run.

Why had it worked? In his previous marathons, where he ran the entire race, giving it all he had every step of the way, he slowed down dramatically in the last 7 miles. However, in this last marathon, he actually picked up his pace in those final miles, shaving 5 minutes off his previous best time in that last stretch, giving him the kick he needed to reach his allegedly unreachable goal.

Let's relate this whole walking business specifically to this program: Take a 1-minute break every 3-5 minutes from the start of each long run. If you feel so inclined, you can run the maximum—5 minutes—between breaks. However, when you reach 18 miles, drop down to a break every 3 minutes.

On to other matters. Note the hill work, commencing with the first Sunday workout. The numbers in parenthesis that follow the hills denote the total mileage, including warm-up, cool-down, the hills themselves, and any other running you might do that day.

Hills play a valuable role in training. They particularly strengthen the calf muscles, and other muscles in the back of the leg, working both primary and secondary running muscles. Thus, hills help the runner shift his weight farther forward on his foot and ankle and lift off more powerfully with each step.

You do the hill work by taking it easy. Warm up slowly for one or two miles. Find a gentle sloping hill, anywhere between 200 to 800 meters in length. Run to the top of the hill, not trying to sprint or exert beyond what is comfortable. Run smoothly, easily, all the way to the top and then over. Walk down the other side.

When running, keep your feet low to the ground while maintaining your upright posture. Keep your stride short, especially at the beginning. As you become more relaxed and capable, you can increase your pace a bit. Whenever the incline increases, or whenever you feel yourself pulling or pushing your legs more than feels right, shorten your stride.

You'll also see a notation on the Sunday schedule listed as 3-4 x 1 mile, 4-5 x 1 mile, and so on. These are called mile repeats, and that's exactly what you do, run a mile, walk between, and do another, all at the prescribed pace. This is a form of interval training, which is done by world-class athletes everywhere. Mile repeats will help you achieve the pace that will carry you to your marathon time goal.

Running fast in the marathon doesn't mean sprinting. Rather, it refers to being able to maintain a moderate pace for considerable distances. In addition, these sessions will teach you how to pace yourself, and how to judge your pace.

It's best if you can train with other people. You can take turns timing each other, and you can turn the mile repeats into run get-togethers. Make no mistake: this can be hard work, so anything you can do to lighten the load is worthwhile. Concentrate on not running too fast, especially in the first few hundred yards. You want to be realistic about your abilities and your goals, and you want the pace on the mile repeats to reflect a realistic approach to the marathon. Consistently running faster than your desired pace will confuse the development of your internal pace clock, as well as increase your fatigue in a cumulative fashion, ultimately hurting your performance in the marathon.

Each mile during a mile repeat session should be run about 20 seconds faster than the pace you wish to set in the marathon, followed by a walk of at least 400 meters. Thus, to reach the 4:40 goal, run the mile repeats in 10:15 each. That should be the pace you'll run between walk breaks during the marathon itself.

One more vital component of marathon training is learning, practicing and implementing what are called acceleration-gliders. Acceleration-gliders (A-G for short) should be used to warm up before hill work, mile repeats and races. Perform A-Gs in the following manner: Keep your legs and body relaxed from start to finish, especially at the beginning. If you can, find a slight downhill to get your momentum going; if you don't have any downhill stretches available, which serve as your accelerating agent, then shorten your stride length, gradually increasing the number of steps you take, picking up your pace, finding a comfortable rhythm. When you reach that comfortable rhythm, let your legs stretch out to a natural length. Once you reach that appropriate, natural speed, just glide, keeping your feet as low as possible, using as little effort as possible. Glide for a distance, anywhere between 50 and 200 meters, and then rest by either jogging or walking between.

A-Gs should become an important part of your running routine, as they help you both fine-tune your running technique and rest your other running muscles.

The 5k races in the schedule are important because they help you get used to the excitement and pressure of racing, and to hitting your mark and meeting your time goals.

You will see that there is flexibility in the total number of minutes that you should run during any given week. The one rule to follow regarding this elasticity: Never increase the total by more than 10% from one week to the next.

3:30 Marathon

The next schedule is designed to help you reach a more ambitious time of 3 hours and 30 minutes. To achieve this, your mile repeats should be run at 7:40—a very brisk pace, by the way. Remember, it is important that you walk, not jog, between mile repeats, in order to give your legs a real chance to rest and recover, from not just this session, but from the cumulative effect of all your training.

If you should find that you simply can't complete all the mile re-

3:30 Marathon

Weeks 1 – 29

	Mon	Tues	Wed	Thurs	Fri	Sat	Sun
1	XT	40–60	20–30	XT	40–60	off	4–6 hills (5–7 miles)
2	XT	40–60	20–30	XT	40–60	off	5k race (6–7 miles)
3	XT	40–60	20–30	XT	40–60	off	7–8 hills (7–8 miles)
4	XT	40–60	20–30	XT	40–60	off	9–10 hills (8–9 miles)
5	XT	45–60	25–35	XT	45–60	off	5k race (9–10 miles)
6	XT	45–60	25–35	XT	45–60	off	3–5 x 1 mile (12 miles)
7	XT	45–60	25–35	XT	45–60	off	5k race (8 miles)
8	XT	45–60	25–35	XT	45–60	off	6–8 x 1 mile (14 miles)
9	XT	45–60	25–35	XT	45–65	off	5k race (8 miles)
10	XT	45–65	25–40	XT	45–65	off	15–16 miles easy
11	XT	45–65	25–40	XT	45–65	off	5k race (9 miles)
12	XT	45–65	25–40	XT	45–65	off	17–18 miles easy
13	XT	45–65	25–40	XT	45–65	off	7–9 x 1 mile
14	XT	45–65	25–40	XT	45–65	off	19–20 miles easy
15	XT	45–65	25–40	XT	45–65	off	5k race (10 miles)
16	XT	45–65	25–40	XT	45–65	off	8–10 x 1 mile
17	XT	45–65	25–40	XT	45–65	off	22–23 miles easy
18	XT	45–65	25–40	XT	45–65	off	5k race
19	XT	45–65	25–40	XT	45–65	off	5–7 x 1 mile
20	XT	45–65	25–40	XT	45–65	off	25–26 miles easy
21	XT	45–65	25–40	XT	45–65	off	5k race
22	XT	45–65	25–40	XT	45–65	off	4–6 x 1 mile
23	XT	45–65	25–40	XT	45–65	off	28–29 miles easy
24	XT	45–55	25–40	XT	45–65	off	5k or 4 x 1 mile
25	XT	40–45	20–25	XT	40–45	off	4–5 x 1 mile
26	run 40	off	run 30	off	run 30	off	THE MARATHON
27	walk 45	run/walk 30	walk 30–60	run/walk 45	walk 30–60	off	7–10 miles walk–run
28	walk 45	run/walk 45	walk 30–60	run/walk 45	walk 30–60	off	9–15 miles run/walk
29	walk 45	run/walk 45	walk 30–60	run/walk 45	walk 30–60	off	12–20 miles run/walk

peats, or maintain the pace, perhaps your ambitions exceed your reach—at least for now. Other, less drastic, explanations also should be considered: 1) maybe you simply started out faster than you should have; 2) you're still tired from your other training sessions, which means you need more days off, or easier days; 3) you need to do more walking between your mile repeats.

2:39 Marathon

Last but not least, we present the schedule for a marathon that leaves you with a time just under 2 hours and 40 minutes—2:39, to be exact. That constitutes a truly terrific time, an amazing time, a time that precious few of us could ever hope to achieve. Yet here it is, the keys to that rarefied kingdom — if you have the God-given ability, the carefully cultivated skill and the intense, inner drive.

What is fascinating is how similar this schedule is to all the others. Cross training, walking combined with running, hill work, 5k races, mile repeats, even a day off — it's not dissimilar in philosophy from the other marathon training programs at all. Of course, the mile repeats should be run at a clip of 5:40 per mile, which is a pace reserved for the truly fleet of foot.

However, pace is not the basic issue here. Instead, what counts is this: Whether you're breaking records or barely breaking a sweat, running, at its essence is a wonderful, liberating activity.

Set your goals and go . . .

2:39 Marathon

Weeks 1 – 29

	Mon	Tues	Wed	Thurs	Fri	Sat	Sun
1	XT or 3 easy	40–55	20–50	XT	40–55	off	4–6 hills (5–7 miles)
2	XT or 3 easy	40–60	20–50	XT	40–60	off	5k race (6–7 miles)
3	XT or 3 easy	40–65	20–50	XT	40–60	off	7–8 hills (7–8 miles)
4	XT or 3 easy	40–65	20–50	XT	40–60	off	9–10 hills (8–9 miles)
5	XT or 3 easy	45–75	25–55	XT	45–65	off	5k race (9–10 miles)
6	XT or 3 easy	45–80	25–55	XT	45–65	off	5–7 x 1 mile (11 miles)
7	XT or 3 easy	45–80	25–55	XT	45–70	off	5k race (8 miles)
8	XT or 4 easy	45–80	25–55	XT	45–75	off	6–8 x 1 mile (13 miles)
9	XT or 4 easy	45–80	25–55	XT	45–80	off	8–10 x 1 mile (12 miles)
10	XT or 4 easy	45–85	25–60	XT	45–85	off	15–16 miles easy
11	XT or 4 easy	45–85	25–60	XT	45–85	off	5k race (9 miles)
12	XT or 4 easy	45–85	25–60	XT	45–85	off	17–18 miles easy
13	XT or 4 easy	45–85	25–60	XT	45–85	off	10–11 x 1 mile
14	XT or 4 easy	45–85	25–60	XT	45–85	off	19–20 miles easy
15	XT or 4 easy	45–85	25–60	XT	45–85	off	5k race (10 miles)
16	XT or 4 easy	45–85	25–60	XT	45–85	off	11–13 x 1 mile
17	XT or 4 easy	45–85	25–60	XT	45–85	off	22–23 miles easy
18	XT or 4 easy	45–85	25–60	XT	45–85	off	5k race
19	XT or 4 easy	45–85	25–60	XT	45–85	off	5–8 x 1 mile
20	XT or 4 easy	45–85	25–60	XT	45–85	off	25–26 miles easy
21	XT or 4 easy	45–85	25–60	XT	45–85	off	5k race
22	XT or 4 easy	45–85	25–60	XT	45–85	off	5–8 x 1 mile
23	XT or 4 easy	45–75	25–60	XT	45–75	off	28–30 miles easy
24	XT	45–55	25–50	XT	45–55	off	5k or 4 x 1 mile
25	XT	40	20–35	XT	40	off	4–6 x 1 mile
26	run 40	off	run 30	off	run 30	off	**THE MARATHON**
27	walk 45	run/walk 40	XT 30–60	run/walk 40	XT 30–60	off	7–10 miles walk–run
28	walk 45	run/walk 45	XT 30–60	run/walk 45	XT 30–60	off	9–15 miles run/walk
29	walk 45	run/walk 45	XT 30–60	run/walk 45	XT 30–60	off	12–20 miles run/walk

CHAPTER 9

Nutrition and Diet

PROPER NUTRITION IS VITAL to any health and fitness program. In this chapter Stephanie Jenkins, a certified nutritionist with a degree in exercise physiology, provides some important advice on nutrition and diet. Stephanie has experience in every aspect of the fitness industry, from developing wellness centers for health clubs to serving as a nutritionist for athletes competing in the Olympic trials and Pan Am Games, to working with hundreds of private clients, to writing a nutrition and wellness column for the *Los Angeles Times*.

It's a safe bet that many of you are interested in treadmill training because you want to lose weight. Sure, it's nice to have muscles, breathe easier, feel good and all the rest, but hey what we really want is to fit into those pants!

There's no getting around it: to lose weight you have to be active. Dieting alone won't do it. In fact, the vast majority of people who use diet alone to lose weight eventually fail, and fail

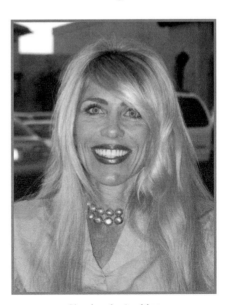

Stephanie Jenkins

badly; most not only gain back the weight, but actually add on a few more pounds. The ultimate insult to injury, you might say.

The fact is neither dieting nor exercising alone leads to successful, permanent weight loss. The key is to combine exercise and dietary changes to result in the greatest amount of weight and fat loss. When dieters also exercise, they lose more pounds and body fat than those who only cut calories. They also maintain their weight loss for longer periods. The reason is clear: Exercise builds muscle tissue, and more muscle allows your body to burn more calories all the time — even when you are resting! Thus, the more muscle you have, the more energy you burn.

This rate of burning up fat is what metabolism is all about. The higher your metabolic rate, the more calories you can consume, while remaining leaner. And, nothing speeds up your metabolism or shifts it into higher gear, better than exercise.

A few statistics: There are 3,500 calories in one pound of body weight. To shed one pound, you must take in 3,500 fewer calories than you expend; to gain that pound, you must take in 3,500 more calories than you use. On the average, a deficit or excess of 500 calories a day brings about a weight loss or gain or about one pound a week. Based on that calculation, an excess or deficit of 1,000 calories a day will result in a change, plus or minus, of two pounds per week.

These numbers are not hard and fast. Many factors can have an impact on them. You may possess an unusually active metabolism, or an extra sluggish one. You may have hormonal imbalances. Trauma and stress can alter your body's response to metabolic function, and therefore affect weight gain and loss.

All of these factors can cause abnormal weight shifts. Regardless, as a rule of thumb, most people can maintain an energy balance with proper eating habits and regular exercise.

And so we move on to what is really important in the weight loss business, and that means body fat. Even more important than weighing yourself, and judging your success and failure by what the scale announces, is calculating the percentage of body fat and lean muscle that you possess.

Stated again: the critical factor in attaining a healthy weight is not how many pounds you weigh, but the percentage of body fat that you are carrying around.

A pound or two, up or down, does not necessarily indicate body fat gained or lost, and it is body fat reduction that will ultimately make a difference in your appearance.

In fact, losing weight quickly by starving yourself, even following the latest popular diet, will result in the loss of lean muscle mass, not fat deposits, and increase your percentage of body fat by slowing down your metabolism. In other words, though you might be lighter in total poundage, you will actually be fatter, in terms of body fat percentage.

That means that a person who doesn't seem to weigh much at all may actually be overly "fat" in terms of body fat, while a person who weighs more and is larger, by all appearances, may be in terrific condition and have less fat. Serious athletes with well-developed muscles and dense bones may actually be heavier, according to the scale, but appear to be quite thin.

The conditioned body is "trained" to use fatty acids, rather than glucose, as fuel. This means that as you become more conditioned, you will tend to burn more body fat during exercise, as well as afterwards, than you did before. The best kind of exercise for building up your fat-burning metabolism is not severely strenuous, but moderate exercise of long duration, which means a minimum of 30-40 minutes, 3 to 5 times per week. Moderate exercise will stimulate your metabolism up to five percent above your normal rate, for as long as two days after the exercise is completed.

Given the importance of understanding body fat, it might be advisable to test your percentage of body fat (see chart on page 110) to determine if you need to lose fat. Many health clubs or sports medicine clinics offer such tests. Once you know your body fat percentage, focus on reducing your measurements and inches rather than your scale weight.

* * *

Just for fun—probably the wrong term, considering what we're talking about—here are a few examples of foods and their calories, and how long you must walk or run to work them off. Of course, these figures are only approximations, and depend on many things, from you body weight to the size of the portion.

Food	Walking	Running
Beer or cola, 12 oz. (150 calories)	58 min.	16 min.
T-bone steak, 8 oz. (800 calories)	5 hrs.	1-1/2 hrs.
Cheese pizza, 1 slice (300 calories)	2 hrs.	33 min.
Chocolate chip cookie (50 calories)	20 min.	5 min.
Ice cream, 2/3 cup (200 calories)	76 min.	22 min.

As you can see, it is easy to add up calories rapidly, and not as easy to burn them off. This is why you might want to take a second to choose foods wisely, and try not to eat too many "empty" foods with low nutrient values and high fat content.

• • •

Since we broached the subject of nutritional value in some foods, let's continue on along this track, and talk about some proper diet hints for athletes.

As an overall rule, a variety of nutrient-dense foods offers the best source of nutrition for those athletically inclined. Contrary to what diet books tell you, no single diet can deliver that long-sought magic bullet, the elixir that suits any or all athletes' bodies perfectly, that raises performance to its peak. It just doesn't work that way, not in the real world.

Nonetheless . . .

Start with unprocessed foods. Concentrate on eating foods that haven't been enhanced with chemicals, dosed with sugar, stuffed with saturated fats, and otherwise treated, preserved and altered. Naturally nutrient-dense foods are the foods that supply maximum vitamins and minerals for the energy they provide. They include fresh fruits and vegetables (cooked as little as possible), as well as quality proteins with low amounts of fats, whole grains, and a small amount of the right kinds of fats, such as olive oil and canola oil.

Processed foods suffer nutrient losses, even when fortified or enriched. Manufactured additives cannot compensate for the whole range of nutrients (and non-nutrients) lost in the processing process. What nature has brought together, let no man tear asunder.

One simple example: processing often removes magnesium and chromium from foods; processing cannot put these essential minerals back into those tampered foods.

Foods that are of lesser benefit to the athlete are white flour products, cheeses, red meat, refined sugar products, soft drinks, fried foods, fast foods, and our old friend, processed foods. These foods will uniformly fill you with lots of calories, without the nutrients, vitamins and minerals you require. They will not enhance your athletic performance, or performance of any sort.

To many this will sound as though there is an implied choice: good food (meaning healthy) corresponds with bad taste (meaning bland). Is this so? Is the issue this black and white? Or are there gradations, where a food—a real food, a popular, delicious, not-on-any-diet-you-heard-of food, can line up nutrients and taste on the side of the angels?

Yes. It all depends on how wisely you select the origin of that food. For instance, take pizza, as so many of would love to do, over and over, day in, day out. You can rest assured that if you buy it from a fast-food chain, the odds are that the unhealthy quotient, from fat to grease to preservatives to who knows what, will border on frightening. But if you have pizza that is prepared with the freshest ingredients, fresh tomato, light on the cheese and with just a bit of olive oil, then it becomes a far healthier dish.

When it comes to your own food, choose healthy versions of favorite foods by using fresh, wholesome ingredients.

• • •

The charts on page 111 give examples of foods that contain the most vitamins and minerals, essential to optimal health and fitness. They are broken into three categories: complex carbohydrates, which should make up 55 to 65% of your daily consumption, proteins, accounting for 15 to 20% of that daily total, and fats, kicking in at 20 to 25% of total calories. (The percentage in each category may vary depending upon the type of athlete you are, and the type of fitness results you wish to obtain. However, for the average exerciser, these percentages are a safe bet.)

Don't forget to drink water, and lots of it, at least eight glasses per day. Water is not only essential to forestall dehydration, cramps and heat stroke, it's also good for your digestion and your skin.

Body Fat Percentage Categories

	Women	Men
Essential fat	10 – 12%	2 – 4%
Athletic	14 – 20%	6 – 13%
Fit	21 – 24%	14 – 17%
Acceptable	25 – 31%	18 – 25%
Obese	>31%	>25%

Source: American Council on Exercise, Personal Trainer Manual, 1997

Female athletes should be careful not to become deficient in iron. Strenuous exercise can deplete iron, and thus cause anemia. It is not a bad idea to periodically have your blood tested to check mineral levels.

Remember, these are just suggestions, just guidelines. Don't throw away your walnut chunk cookies. Don't throw away your mint chocolate fudge.

Just try to put them down every now and then.

Eating counts. Nutrition counts. Beyond eating for survival, athletes—and don't forget, that includes you—must eat for energy, and energy requirements can be intense. The more you exercise, the more you need to eat in a healthy manner.

If you happen to be the type who is inclined to become a bit obsessive about calories and fat and fiber, etc., don't drive yourself crazy. On the other hand, if you're going to go to the trouble of exercising, working hard to get into the best shape you can attain (or at least better shape than you currently are in), why not cut down on the ways you sabotage all your effort and sweat?

Just a little food for thought.

Complex Carbohydrates — 55 to 65 % daily total

tomatoes	broccoli
cabbage	kale
cauliflower	carrots
green, leafy vegetables	onions
garlic	asparagus
blueberries	strawberries
apples	watermelons
oranges	grapefruits
pineapples	apricots
papaya	bananas
cantaloupe	whole grain breads
brown rice	potatoes
whole grain cereals	

Proteins — 15 to 20 % daily total

fresh fish (salmon, mackerel, tuna, halibut)	chicken
turkey	low/nonfat yogurt
low/nonfat milk	low/nonfat cottage cheese
soy products	nuts and seeds
beans	

Fats — 20 to 25 % daily total

monosaturated and polyunsaturated fats	olive oil
canola oil	flaxseed oil
fish oils	avocado

CHAPTER 10

When You're Ready to Buy a Treadmill

NOW THAT YOU'RE READY TO GO out and buy a treadmill (or seriously thinking about it), let's talk about what you should know.

The first factor to consider is how you intend to use the machine. Buying a treadmill is not different from buying anything else: Buy what you need, no more, no less. Just as you wouldn't buy an Armani suit to do your gardening, you shouldn't buy a treadmill designed for Olympic sprinters if you just plan to walk on it while reading the Wall Street Journal.

At the same time, you want to ensure that you haven't shortchanged yourself by purchasing a treadmill that isn't adequate for both your needs and your safety. You might not be a world-class sprinter, but you require an unfailingly smooth track as much as any track star. Maybe you aren't burning up the tread with sub five-minute miles; nonetheless, your treadmill had better accelerate and decelerate without a hitch. Regardless of your training level, and of how long or how fast you run, everybody, from beginner to expert, needs to work out on a treadmill that is reliable and comfortable.

An under-powered, unstable or flimsy machine can cause injury through unpredictable performance. Even if you don't suffer some harm, the experience might be so disheartening that you abandon treadmill training altogether. After all, the point is to enjoy your workouts, to look forward to your sessions and relish your training time. Hopefully, you'll regard your exercise as fun. Even if that's too optimistic, and you'll never be transformed into a happy devotee of the sweating set, at the very least you must have a treadmill that makes your daily or thrice-weekly encounter as painless and as untroubled as possible.

The truth is, the most common reason that people stop going to the gym, whether that gym is across town or in their spare bedroom, is that it is too much of a hassle. There might be too few parking spots or crowded work stations. Most likely, those people simply do not enjoy the act of exercising. The right gym and/or the right equipment can make all the difference in the world, both physically and psychologically. And when you're giving it all you've got — or even giving it a certain percentage of what you're capable of — the psychological part can be more consequential than the physical.

Here are some simple and practical guidelines for purchasing a treadmill:

• Steel is stronger than aluminum, and welds are stronger than rivets or bolts. The stronger the frame material and construction, the more solid and dependable the machine.

• The treadmill you pick should have easy-to-read and equally easy-to-use control panels. That adds up to large numeric displays, intelligently and simply organized selection buttons, and straightforward programming. Operation then becomes virtually intuitive for the runner.

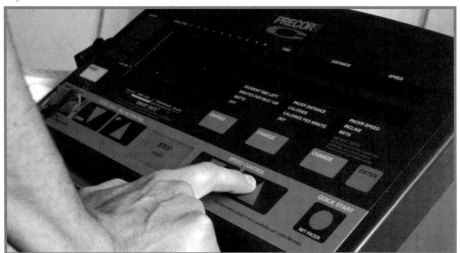

- In the same vein, the book containing the operating instructions should be user-friendly.
- The cushioning on the track should be substantial. However, it should absorb the shock of your impact without rebounding like a trampoline.
- The ability of the machine to elevate should be electronic, not manual, and the operation should be absolutely smooth, so there is no problem raising or lowering the treadmill while running.
- Widths and lengths of treadmills widely vary; make certain any treadmill you are considering has sufficient width and length for you to feel comfortable. Turn on the machine in the store full-bore, so you can hear how much noise it produces and how much it vibrates. Raise and lower it at the same time, adding in the noise and vibration from that separate motor as well. (The noise level might not seem so important standing in the store, but wait till you get it home, and you can't hear the television over the treadmill's motor, and your children complain they can't study over the tumult. Actually, you should be so lucky, at least as far as the latter example is concerned.)

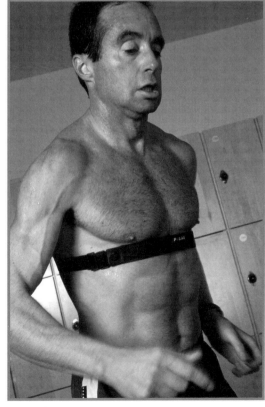

- Check to see what sort of programmed workouts the machine has, if programs are a feature you will use.
- If you want a heart monitor, make sure the machine has one. Wireless heart monitors that strap around your chest are the best, those that have you grab onto the handrails are also good. The least effective are the sensors mounted on the console that you touch with your thumb.

- An emergency shut-off button or key is a necessity, and is standard on any decent machine.
- Don't dismiss the aesthetics of the machine — after all, you're going to share your home with it. To some, the style and shape of the machine is important. Others don't care. Where do you stand? On another issue, do you find the console welcoming? Does it have a space or compartment for a water bottle or TV remote — and does that matter to you?
- Though a treadmill should be an extremely dependable machine, absent any troubles for many years, read the warranty carefully so you are confident that the company will stand behind it, come what may.

Finally, and perhaps most obviously, before buying any machine, try it out. Whatever you do, don't buy a treadmill over the phone after watching an infomercial at 2 a.m. Go to a retail outlet or seek out a well-equipped gym, kick the tires, check under the hood, and take it

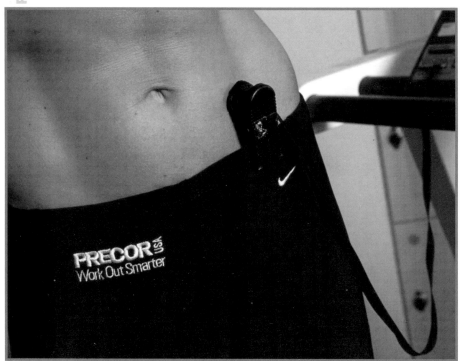

Precor Treadmills include a clip-on emergency shut off key.

out for a test drive. Don't go to just any store, select one that specializes in athletic equipment, preferably high-end athletic equipment, rather than a department store that sells everything under the sun — plus treadmills. Why? Because specialty stores sell better quality, more reliable, and more efficient equipment, and usually are staffed by sales personnel who actually know something about what they are selling. If you want to buy shoes that actually fit, you go to a shoe store that has somebody who knows how to measure your foot and help you select the right shoe for you. If you're looking for flip-flops to kick around on the beach for a few weeks, you stop in at the local drug store and pick a pair for ninety-nine cents out of a giant bin filled with flip-flops of all sizes and colors.

A Treadmill is not a Flip-Flop.

Precor only sells its treadmills and other machines in stores that specialize in better athletic equipment because it wants its customers to have the best opportunity to get exactly what they want when they decide to purchase a treadmill.

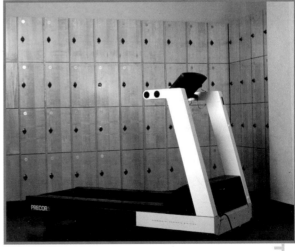

Take your time when you try out the machine, and ask yourself—and whoever else is around—any questions that come to mind. Does the treadmill feel comfortable? Does it fit you, in some intangible way? In a much more tangible way, does it fit the space you intend to be its new home? Is it truly the machine for you?

In the same way that you want to exercise "smart," shop "smart" for your treadmill and you won't be disappointed.

CHAPTER 11

Work Out Smarter

THIS BOOK IS DESIGNED to serve two purposes. First, it intends to be a forthright, practical account of how you can start or improve a walking or running program. It also seeks to inspire you through the life examples and philosophies of running experts.

While we have covered many topics, there is much more to say, many more possibilities to consider. As you step onto your treadmill and begin to determine exactly how much time and effort you are willing expend, and as you discover what you want to accomplish, you will take the ideas and programs in this book and expand upon them. You will discover your own path to the perfect exercise routine for you.

And make no mistake, that perfect routine is not static or permanent. Most likely, your training schedule will continue to evolve as you evolve; as your age, your weight, and your muscle mass change, and as your perceptions and goals change.

Implicit in these words is that there are no exercise miracles or panaceas. Yes, exercise is important and good. Yes, you can change your body, your health and your life. Those changes are attainable, and within a relatively short time frame. However, nothing can be achieved without effort and determination. And the treadmill can't achieve your goals for you, only you can do that.

Not only must you take the initiative and start training, you must be the manager of your training. That means that you have to be acutely aware of your progress, and alter your training whenever necessary to adjust for shifting goals, injuries or situations.

There is a world of possibility for you—you just need to choose to act.

As you evolve personally, technology will also keep changing, and improving, as will information and understanding about how the body responds and works. The programs and machines to include in your exercise program are your choices. As you grow more familiar with training and scheduling, you will be better equipped to make well-informed judgments.

The treadmill can't achieve your goals for you, only you can do that.

As we noted in the very first chapter, Precor calls this approach—the creation and maintenance of a system of ongoing improvement, of unending innovation—"Work Out Smarter."

Whether talking about the needs and goals of an individual or a corporation, that's not a bad philosophy.

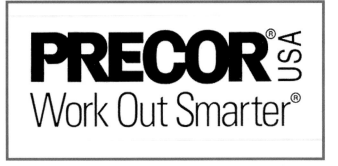

EPILOGUE

Alberto's Final Say

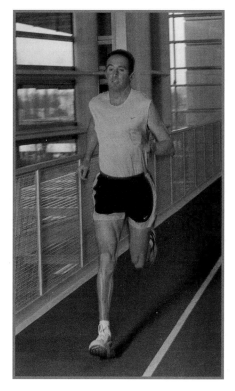

WE'VE REACHED THE END OF THE BOOK and it's time to step back and reflect not just on what we've learned, but also on where we're going. After all, you've been presented with a ton of information—so what's next?

Of course, the answer is different for each one of us. I'm going to tell you what it is for me. I opened the book by talking about the past, about the beginning of my career. Now I'd like to talk about my future.

As the 2000 Olympic Games in Sydney draw near, I've been thinking about how long ago I was running at a world-class level, and wondering whether I can reach that competitive rank again. I still aspire to qualify for the U.S. Olympic Marathon Trials, as well as to successfully compete in ultra events (ultra defined as anything longer than marathon distance).

I'm 41 years old. No matter how you figure it, no matter how hard or long you train, two score and some change means I'm past my physical prime.

This is not to say that I'm on the way to obsolescence. I still work out diligently and strenuously, and consider myself to be in good shape. However, when you're talking about competing at the world-class level, no amount of training can fully compensate for the passing of time. And when you consider time, you have to consider injuries. I've had my share of injuries, and they take not only an immediate toll, but a cumulative one as well.

The last competitive marathon I ran was the 1984 Olympic Marathon, and I finished a disappointing fifteenth. I know I have a long mountain to climb if I want to compete at what I would judge a respectable level.

On the other hand, there are a couple of things working in my favor. Intellectually, I am better prepared than ever to get the most from my training. I have a more thorough grasp of the mechanics of exercise and physiology than at any other point in my career. I also have a finer appreciation of my capabilities, and a more honest and reasonable perspective of what place running has in my life. As a result, I am mentally stronger now than when I was younger.

In 1994, I won the Comrades Ultra Marathon, the most prestigious ultra-distance race in the world, a race rich in history, like the Boston Marathon. The 54-mile event attracts some 15,000 men and women every year.

As I mentioned in the prologue, shortly after this victory I ruptured a tendon while training. Since then I have had ten surgeries on my foot and leg, culminating in a total foot reconstruction nine months ago.

Despite this setback, I'm now close to my best condition, running up to 100 miles a week. My goal is to race again, with an emphasis on ultra-distance events. At my age, I feel I still have the physical talent, and the mental and emotional disposition to rank among the best in the world at ultra distances, which are ordinarily twice that of a marathon.

I figure that I've probably lost the speed to compete in the marathon on the world stage, where the pace is well under 5 minutes per mile. At the same time, I know I can handle the pace for an ultra marathon.

My confidence stems in large part from the intellectual insight and mental toughness mentioned above, which translates into knowing how to best train. That's where the treadmill comes in. It's as useful a tool as you can find, both for getting fit and avoiding injury. Back in 1994, when I was training for the Comrades Ultra, I did half my weekly 120 miles on the treadmill, which left me both ready and healthy.

Much of what I learned, as well as a lot of what some other people know, is found in this book. I am confident that it can help you achieve your fitness goals. I can't guarantee that you will run a particular time. Several factors, from genetics to psychology to how much time your kids or job take away from your athletic endeavors, will influence that.

Set realistic goals—whether they be race times, weight loss or cardiovascular conditioning—that take into account your age, current fitness level and background. If you do, intelligence, patience and determination can guide you to a satisfying, happy result.

Nothing is guaranteed in life. We all know that. Nevertheless, we owe it to ourselves to make the most of our abilities and opportunities, to make the most of ourselves. That includes, at the top of the list, protecting our health and enhancing our physical well-being — and exercise is surely one of the primary ways to do that.

Take what you've learned here, apply it as diligently and as thoughtfully as you can. The healthiest and, perhaps, the best part of your life lies ahead.

Crunch® Fitness Series

Through the country Crunch® is synonymous with the ultimate in fitness and exercise. From New York to LA, Crunch Fitness Centers have helped hundreds of thousands of Americans get in shape and stay in shape. With their unique lifestyle approach to fitness and their philosophy of "no judgements" on your lifestyle, Crunch is the choice of men and women who want to exercise their right to fitness.

Crunch and Hatherleigh are proud to announce the next three books in the *Crunch Fitness Series*. Each book in the series is specifically designed to meet the lifestyle demands of today's Americans — the harried business executive who spends her weekends on the road, the father of the bride who has to look good in a tux, the soccer mom who just doesn't have time for the gym, young people, old people, couch potatoes and bodybuilders.

Everyone will benefit from the Crunch expertise and their team of fitness specialists.

Crunch is a major national chain of fitness centers. Their brand is widely recognized through a daily television exercise show on ESPN and through their videos and fitness apparel. Their upscale, user-friendly gyms are located in New York, Los Angeles, San Francisco, Miami, Chicago, and Tokyo.

Also available in the
Crunch Fitness Series:

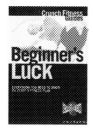 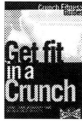 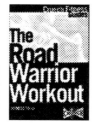

Beginner's Luck
Get Fit in a Crunch
The Road Warrior Workout

Perfect Posture

Mom always told you to stand up straight, and she was right!

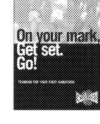

Good posture is very beneficial in a variety of ways — it can make you look better, feel better, and helps relieve a wide range of muscle and spine related complaints. The Crunch Perfect Posture book presents a combination of exercises, stretches and "Americanized" yoga techniques that will lead you to improved posture.

Also included are tips on selecting a mattress, the proper way to sit, how to prevent back injuries, and breathing exercises to help your spine and back.

October 1999 / $14.95 (Can. $20.99) / paper / 120 pages
ISBN 1-57826-040-X / 6 x 9   Diet & Health/Fitness

Workouts for Workaholics

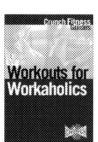

Get your body in shape while you keep you career in gear!

Maintaining fitness on the job will help you work more productively, deal better with physical and emotional stress, and reduce sickness. This book shows you how to find the time at work to keep in shape. Includes exercises that can be done at your desk in business attire, relaxation techniques to fight stress, nutrition tips, and scheduling plans to get you out of the workplace and to a workout with the last amount of disruption.

October 1999 / $14.95 (Can. $20.99) / paper / 120 pages
ISBN 1-57826-041-8 / 6 x 9   Diet & Health/Fitness

On Your Mark. Get Set. Go!
Training for you first marathon.

The marathon is the crown jewel of running. 26.2 miles of exhilaration and sometimes agony. This book is designed to get the novice, recreational runner from the starting line to the finish line. In keeping with Crunch's philosophy, there's no judgement on your finishing time, we just want you to finish. Covers everything to get you in shape mentally and physically including nutrition, detailed training schedules, exercises and stretches, the right equipment, dealing with pain and avoiding injuries.

October 1999 / $14.95 (Can. $20.99) / paper / 120 pages
ISBN 1-57826-050-7 / 6 x 9   Diet & Health/Fitness

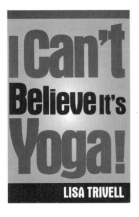

GOLF FLEX:
10 Minutes a Day to Better Play

Wouldn't you like to beat the pants off your golf buddies by adding 60 yards to your drive? How about knocking strokes off your game?

Master trainer and conditioning expert Paul Frediani has developed a scientific program which is guaranteed to make you a better golfer and he calls it *Golf Flex*.

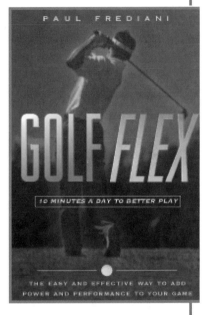

Golf Flex targets your body's power zones and increases your flexibility in these defined areas. The program takes just 10 minutes a day and can be done at your desk, in your car, at home, wherever. Combined with a special pre-game series of stretches, Golf Flex gives you the advantage you've been looking for.

No doubt about it, the pros have added flexibility to their training for years. This closely guarded secret has now become available to golfer's everywhere. Beat your buddies to the punch by picking up your copy of *Golf Flex* today!

Written by Paul Frediani, ACSM

$9.95 ISBN: 1-57826-031-0

The Official Boot Camp Workout presents a total body fitness program combining strength, endurance, flexibility, and cardio-conditioning. From coast to coast, everyone's discovering this "no frills," high energy approach to fitness.

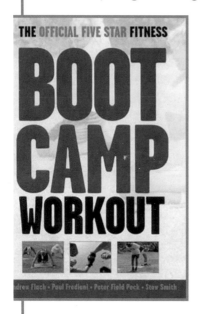

The Official Boot Camp Workout will show you how to build a strong foundation for life-long fitness. Detailed, progressive 6-week workout plans for beginner, intermediate, and advanced workout warriors are featured. Minimal exercise equipment is required.

• • •

Whether you want to get strong, lose weight, increase your energy, or just have a fun workout, **The Official Boot Camp Workout** is the answer!

Written by
Andrew Flach, Paul Frediani, Stew Smith
Photographed by Peter Field Peck

$14.95 ISBN: 1-57826-033-7

Available in bookstores everywhere,
order toll free at 1-800-906-1234
or online at getfitnow.com.